LASIK:
Clinical
Co-Management

LASIK: Clinical Co-Management

Edited by

Milton M. Hom, O.D., F.A.A.O.

Private Practice, Azusa, California

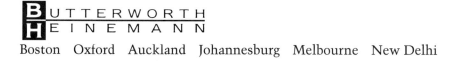

BUTTERWORTH
HEINEMANN

Boston   Oxford   Auckland   Johannesburg   Melbourne   New Delhi

Every effort has been made to ensure that the drug dosage schedules within this text are accurate and conform to standards accepted at time of publication. However, as treatment recommendations vary in the light of continuing research and clinical experience, the reader is advised to verify drug dosage schedules herein with information found on product information sheets. This is especially true in cases of new or infrequently used drugs.

Recognizing the importance of preserving what has been written, Butterworth–Heinemann prints its books on acid-free paper whenever possible.

GLOBAL Butterworth–Heinemann supports the efforts of American Forests and the Global ReLeaf RELEAF program in its campaign for the betterment of trees, forests, and our environment.

Library of Congress Cataloging-in-Publication Data
LASIK : clinical co-management / [edited by] Milton M. Hom.
   p. ; cm.
   Includes bibliographical references and index.
   ISBN 0-7506-7214-5 (alk. paper)
   1. LASIK (Eye surgery) I. Hom, Milton M.
   [DNLM: 1. Keratomileusis, Laser In Situ. WW 220 L3443 2001]
   RE336 .L275 2001
   617.7'55—dc21
                                                                    00-029752

British Library Cataloguing-in-Publication Data
A catalogue record for this book is available from the British Library.

The publisher offers special discounts on bulk orders of this book.
For information, please contact:

Manager of Special Sales
Butterworth–Heinemann
225 Wildwood Avenue
Woburn, MA 01801-2041
Tel: 781-904-2500
Fax: 781-904-2620

For information on all Butterworth–Heinemann publications available, contact our World Wide Web home page at: http://www.bh.com

10 9 8 7 6 5 4 3 2

Printed in the United States of America

This book is dedicated to my family:
Jill, Jennifer, and Zachary Hom;
and to our parents/grandparents:
Milton and Norma Hom and Chester and Katherine Chan.

Contents

Contributing Authors

Michael R. Boland, O.D.
Optometric Director, Excimer Vision Leasing, The Laser Center at Northeastern Eye Institute, Scranton, Pennsylvania

Charlotte Burns, O.D., M.S., F.A.A.O.
Regional Clinical Director, TLC Laser Eye Center, Lodi, Wisconsin

Michael D. DePaolis, O.D., F.A.A.O.
Clinical Associate in Ophthalmology, University of Rochester School of Medicine and Dentistry and Strong Memorial Hospital, Rochester, New York

Arthur B. Epstein, O.D., F.A.A.O.
Clinical Adjunct Assistant Professor, Northeastern State University College of Optometry, Tahlequah, Oklahoma; Director, Contact Lens Service, North Shore University Hospital and New York University School of Medicine, Great Neck, New York

Milton M. Hom, O.D., F.A.A.O.
Private Practice, Azusa, California

Paul M. Karpecki, O.D.
Faculty, Department of Ophthalmology, University of Missouri-Kansas City School of Medicine; Clinical Director of Refractive Surgery, Hunkeler Eye Centers, Kansas City, Missouri

Robert W. Lingua, M.D.
Associate Clinical Professor of Ophthalmology, University of California, Irvine, College of Medicine; Medical Director, TLC The Brea Laser Eye Center, Brea, California

Steven H. Linn, O.D.
Optometric Fellow, Cornea and Refractive Surgery, Hunkeler Eye Centers, Kansas City, Missouri

Robert A. Ryan, O.D.
Adjunct Instructor in Ophthalmology, University of Rochester School of Medicine and Dentistry, New York; Staff Optometrist, Strong Memorial Hospital, Rochester, New York

Joseph P. Shovlin, O.D., F.A.A.O.
Adjunct Clinical Faculty, Pennsylvania College of Optometry, Philadelphia; Senior Optometrist and Director of Refractive Surgery Services, Northeastern Eye Institute, Scranton, Pennsylvania

Loretta B. Szczotka, O.D., M.S., F.A.A.O.
Assistant Professor of Ophthalmology, Case Western Reserve University School of Medicine, Cleveland, Ohio; Director, Contact Lens Service, University Ophthalmologists, Inc., University Hospitals of Cleveland

Preface

Until recently, a book like *LASIK: Clinical Co-Management* would not be possible because the procedure was not prevalent in the United States. I am pleased to have the opportunity to write about LASIK from the optometric point of view.

I would like to thank Jan P. Bergmanson, Kenneth A. Lebow, Bob Lingua, and Arthur B. Epstein for reviewing chapters, and Steven H. Linn for the main cover photo. A special note of thanks to Loretta B. Szczotka for her hard work and support.

Even as this book evolved, the techniques of LASIK were updated and improved. The world of refractive surgery is constantly evolving. The LASIK technique as we know it today will continue to improve as time goes on. On the horizon there are newer and better technologies, as described in Chapter 11 (Future Techniques and Investigational Procedures). In a few years, LASIK may no longer be the primary refractive procedure but one of many procedures available to our patients to correct their ametropias. The role of the optometrist in co-management, however, will always be significant.

MILTON M. HOM

CHAPTER 1

Introduction

Milton M. Hom

> The lamellar surgery goal: a living contact lens without the contact lens regimen or worries.
> —John F. Doane[1]

In 1990, Pallikaris et al. first described laser in situ keratomileusis (LASIK) in the literature.[2] LASIK involves lifting a corneal flap with a micro-keratome and ablating the stromal bed with an excimer laser to achieve refractive change.[3] LASIK is capable of correcting myopia, hyperopia, and astigmatism with minimal pain, rapid recovery of vision, and good refractive stability. It allows for repeated surgery for residual refractive error.[4] In the past, the term *flap and zap* has been coined to describe LASIK.[5]

LASIK offers several advantages over photorefractive keratectomy (PRK). In PRK with surface or transepithelial ablations, or both, Bowman's membrane is lost, whereas LASIK preserves it.[4] The haze normally associated with PRK is greatly lessened in LASIK[5] (see Chapter 2, Corneal Healing). LASIK provides the combination of computer-controlled microprecision ablation with the preservation of epithelium and Bowman's membrane.[6] This results in LASIK's greatest advantage, the improved healing and better reliability of outcomes.

Development of LASIK

> Keratomileusis is the first time in the history of medicine that a body part was removed, remodeled through the dictates of the computer and replaced with improved function.
> —Lee T. Nordan[1]

Although LASIK was first described in 1990, its roots can be found in the development of keratomileusis spanning some 40 years of development.[7] Originally developed by Jose Barraquer of Bogotá, Colombia, keratomileusis involves carving the cornea to correct refractive error. The microkeratome is the instrument of choice to carve the cornea or create a corneal flap or disk.[7,8] Over the years, several variations of keratomileu-

1

sis have been seen (Table 1.1). Myopic and hyperopic corrections have been achieved with cryolathe, planar (non-freeze), and excimer laser techniques.[7]

Excimer laser keratomileusis uses an excimer laser to make the refractive cut. Originally, the laser cut was made on the back of the corneal disk created by the microkeratome. In situ keratomileusis, developed by Luis A. Ruiz, involves making the cut in the stromal bed, not the disk.[7,8] An early version of in situ keratomileusis was automated lamellar keratoplasty. Automated lamellar keratoplasty used a mechanical microkeratome to create both the flap and the refractive cut from the stromal bed, which was an attempt to enhance the reliability of the cut.[7] LASIK combines automated lamellar keratoplasty and laser-assisted in situ keratomileusis. The initial cut is made by an automated microkeratome, and the refractive cut is made by the laser on the stromal bed.

TABLE 1.1
Terminology of Keratomileusis

Term	Definition
Keratomileusis	Procedures that use a microkeratome or other instrument to create a corneal flap or disk as a part of refractive keratoplasty.
Myopic keratomileusis	Keratomileusis to treat myopia.
Hyperopic keratomileusis	Keratomileusis to treat hyperopia.
Cryolathe keratomileusis	Keratomileusis for myopia or hyperopia using a cryolathe to change the curvature of the back of the corneal disk.
Planar nonfreeze keratomileusis	Keratomileusis for myopia or hyperopia using a microkeratome and a set of dies to change the curvature of the back of the disk.
Excimer laser keratomileusis	Keratomileusis using the excimer laser to make the refractive cut on the back of the disk.
In situ keratomileusis	Keratomileusis for myopia with refractive cut made in the corneal stromal bed.
Automated lamellar keratoplasty	Neologism for keratomileusis in situ in which a mechanically propelled microkeratome makes the flap or disk and the refractive cut.
Laser in situ keratomileusis (LASIK)	Useful abbreviation for keratomileusis in situ performed with the excimer laser. May be done with a corneal disk or corneal flap.

Source: Reprinted with permission from GO Waring. Excimer Laser In Situ Keratomileusis (LASIK). In CNJ McGhee, HR Taylor, DS Gatry, et al. (eds), Excimer Lasers in Ophthalmology. Boston: Butterworth–Heinemann, 1997;295.

Advantages and Disadvantages of the Procedure

LASIK is an improvement over past conventional refractive surgery proce-dures. Most ametropias, such as myopia, hyperopia, and astigmatism, can be corrected. The surgeon needs to master only one principal technique to cor-rect most patients. Improving computer algorithms allows the outcomes to be further refined. A large part of the LASIK surgical technique is making the cut. Because the cut is made with an automated microkeratome, there is a lower chance of error than with other techniques. The microkeratome also makes a hinged flap, which is less likely to be lost or damaged. Replacement of the flap after the ablation is also more accurate. The healing time is rapid because Bowman's membrane is left intact (see Chapter 2, Corneal Healing). The entire central cornea remains intact, allowing vision to recover quickly. This offers much improvement over PRK, which required a corneal healing time of 3–5 days for clear vision to return. Finally, the ability to retreat or enhance is a distinct advantage. The flap can be lifted at a later time if an enhancement is needed to correct residual refractive error[7] (see Chapter 6, Description of Primary Procedure and Retreatment).

There are several disadvantages of the procedure. The main disadvan-tage is the surgical complications that can occur when creating the flap and handling the microkeratome (see Chapters 6, Description of Primary Proce-dure and Retreatment, and 8, LASIK Complications and Management). The surgeon also does not have control of the laser during the ablation. The com-puter and its algorithms determine the nature of the ablation for a particular target correction. The excimer laser itself is expensive and has hefty mainte-nance costs. Although the procedure is more accurate than previous conven-tional methods of refractive surgery, enhancements are still needed[7] (see Chapter 9, Outcomes). Patient symptoms of halos, glare, and night vision problems need to be addressed. Dry eyes after the procedure are another common problem seen during optometric follow-up. Despite these disad-vantages, LASIK is believed to be the best of the known surgical techniques for correcting myopia and hyperopia with and without astigmatism.[9]

References

1. Doane JF. Building a LASIK Nomogram. In SG Slade (ed), Eyelearn LASIK (vol-ume II). Santa Monica, CA: Digital Interactive Computerized Education, Inc., 1997.
2. Pallikaris IG, Papatzanaki ME, Stathi EZ, et al. Laser in situ keratomileusis. Lasers Surg Med 1990;10:463–468.
3. Perez-Santonja JJ, Bellot J, Claramonte P, et al. Laser in situ keratomileusis to correct high myopia. J Cataract Refract Surg 1997;23:372–385.
4. Lingua RW (ed). The Essentials of LASIK and Its Co-management. Brea, Cali-fornia: TLC Laser Center, 1997.

5. Pallikaris IG, Siganos DS. Laser in situ keratomileusis to treat myopia: early experience. J Cataract Refract Surg 1997;23:39–49.
6. El Danasoruy MA, Waring GO, El Maghraby A, et al. Excimer laser in situ keratomileusis to correct compound myopic astigmatism. J Refract Surg 1997;13:511–520.
7. Waring GO. Excimer Laser In Situ Keratomileusis (LASIK). In CNJ McGhee, HR Taylor, DS Gatry, et al. (eds), Excimer Lasers in Ophthalmology. Boston: Butterworth–Heinemann, 1997.
8. Arbelaez MC, Rapoza PA, Vidaurri-Leal J. LASIK Surgical Techniques. In JH Talamo, RR Krueger (eds), The Excimer Manual: A Clinican's Guide to Excimer Laser Surgery. Boston: Little, Brown, 1997.
9. Guell JL. Experience with laser in situ keratomileusis. J Cataract Refract Surg 1996;22:1391.

CHAPTER 2

Corneal Healing

Milton M. Hom

The cornea undergoes many changes after laser refractive surgery. Most of these changes are related to the healing process. The purpose of this chapter is to review the healing processes to help the practitioner better understand what is occurring when co-managing laser refractive surgery patients. There are several factors involved in corneal healing after the procedure.

Symptoms

When the cornea is wounded, patients usually report varying degrees of pain, photophobia, tearing, foreign body sensation, and sometimes decreased visual acuity.[1] After the microkeratome cut in LASIK and replacement of the flap, the healing process begins. Any pain the patient may experience is generally within 24 hours of the procedure. The patients report symptoms related to corneal wound healing during this time. Immediately after the procedure, the patient typically does not report symptoms because of the anesthesia or anti-anxiety medications administered before the procedure. If there is extreme pain after the procedure, then the flap or epithelium may have been disrupted.[2] As compared to other forms of laser refractive surgery, with LASIK an initial decrease in visual acuity is not a severe problem because most of the corneal surface area is left intact.

Tear Film

Not only is the cornea involved in the healing process, but the tear film also plays a major role. An intact tear film is critical to allowing the cornea to heal properly, and poor tear quality can compromise the wound healing process.[3] The tear film contributes many necessary healing factors, such as defensins platelet-derived growth factor, epidermal growth factor, and transforming growth factor alpha.[4]

After the procedure, the tear film coverage of the cornea is commonly affected. Because of the corneal altered geometry, a break-up of the tear flow over the junctional knee can sometimes be seen. This is usually accompanied by dry eyes. Normally, the symptoms resolve after 1–2 months. Aggressive lubrication is commonly prescribed. Punctal plugs are used for the more severe cases (see Chapter 7, Post-Procedure Management).

Corneal Wound Healing

Wound healing consists of a series of events controlled by many factors. With corneal wounding, there is a communication loss between cells, which initiates the activation of numerous proteins, growth factors, and cellular elements. Much of the same activity that occurred during early corneal development is reactivated.[4] Typically, wound healing ends with scar formation and vascularization. If occurring in the cornea, scar formation and vascularization are unwanted because of the detrimental effects on vision. The ideal wound healing pattern in the cornea results in no scarring or vascularization. The preferred corneal healing pattern would be for the epithelium to perfectly adhere to the stroma and retain its normal thickness. The stroma should have no scarring or regeneration and maintain mechanical stability. The endothelium should also remain unaffected.[3]

With laser refractive surgery, irregularities in healing create focal epithelial hyperplasia, topographic irregularities, and subsequent enhancement problems. As opposed to photorefractive keratectomy (PRK), in LASIK, many of the healing complications are reduced in scope and nature. Focal hyperplasia is not commonly seen with LASIK, because the wound healing is usually isolated to the microkeratome cut and Bowman's membrane is left unaltered.

Pearl:
The ideal corneal wound healing pattern results in no scar formation or vascularization.

Epithelial Healing

With an intact basement membrane (Bowman's membrane), a simple corneal abrasion involves epithelial migration taking place over 2–3 days, followed by thickening of the layers. When the basement membrane is lost (as in PRK), reepithelialization takes place in 5–7 days.[4]

Wound healing is size-dependent. The size of the wound influences the rate of healing. A small wound heals at a slower rate, whereas a large wound heals at a faster rate.[4] For LASIK, the wound heals quickly because the epithelial area damaged is extremely small. Epithelial healing is usually described in four stages: latent phase, cell migration, cell proliferation, and adhesion.

Latent Phase

In the first stage, the latent phase, the cornea prepares itself to close the wound. An extensive cellular and subcellular reorganization takes place at the edge of the wound.[5] Initially, polymorphonuclear leukocytes from the tear layer remove necrotic cells and debris.[3,4,6] The cells at the leading edge of the epithelium are transformed from a stratified, squamous epithelium to a single layer of motile cells.[5] The epithelial cells at the wound's edges lose surface microvilli and subsequently flatten and separate. The hemidesmosomal attachments between the basal cells and basal lamina disappear, allowing the cells to slide.

The latent phase ends with the appearance of cellular processes on the basal edges of the cells bordering the wound. These processes are finger-like filopodia or wider lamellipodia.[3]

Cell Migration

In the second stage, cell migration, cells migrate laterally across the wound area. Four to 6 hours after corneal débridement, the basal epithelial cells slide and move, characterizing the cell migration stage of healing. A monolayer over the wound is created, accounting for the disappearance of most symptoms 4–6 hours after LASIK.[4] The epithelium slides to cover the gutter surrounding the microkeratome cut.

Pearl:
Most of the symptoms after LASIK disappear 4–6 hours after the procedure.

This type of healing is called *linear cell healing*. The cells migrate in a line. Normally, the epithelial cells are attached to the basement membrane with anchoring filaments and desmosomes.[7] A subepithelial matrix of adhesive glycoproteins, fibronectin, and laminin helps to attach the cells to the basement membrane. This subepithelial matrix is located between the basal epithelial cells and the basement membrane and forms a part of the extracellular matrix. A keratin meshwork, basement membrane, proteolytic enzymes, and many growth factors are located in the extracellular matrix.[4]

The main matrix proteins, fibronectin, tenascin, and laminin, play an important role in epithelial healing. For the cells to slide across the wound, the fibronectin and laminin subepithelial matrix needs to be broken.

Greater amounts of fibronectin are synthesized during wound healing.[4] Fibronectin stimulates production of a urokinase-like plasminogen activator that converts plasmogen into plasmin.[7] The plasmin breaks down adhesion between cells and the subepithelial matrix, allowing the cells to slide.[8] The filopodia and lamellipodia bind with and cleave with the subepithelial matrix.

Because the hemidesmosome attachments are disabled, the cells need some sort of support structure as they slide across the wound. Actin filaments, located in the filopodia and lamellipodia, act as cytoskeletal support for the cells as they migrate. The cells attach themselves to the actin filament support structure with the interim adhesion junctions known as *focal adhesions* or *focal contacts*. Fibronectin, vinculin, and actin form focal adhesions.[4]

The regenerated epithelial cells involved in wound response have fibronectin receptors. Fibronectin also causes these newly formed epithelial cells to spread. Normal epithelial cells do not have receptors for fibronectin.[9]

The normal pathway of cell migration is inward, from the limbus to the central cornea in a centripetal fashion, after wounding. The centripetal sheet movement comes from several directions, meeting in an X- or Y-shaped junction as the wound closes.[3,4] The cells migrate as a continuous sheet, with the individual cells maintaining the same relative position to each other. Sometimes, whorls are formed when a column of cells migrates independently.[3]

Cell Proliferation

In the third stage, cell proliferation, the epithelial cells enter a phase of prolific reproduction.[1] Once there is coverage, the epithelial layer is thickened with cell proliferation. Near the limbus are stem cells. The stem cells are responsible for cell replacement and regeneration.[3]

There are two types of epithelial cells: basal cells and overlying suprabasal cells. The stem cells first produce transient amplifying cells. The transient amplifying cells rapidly divide and become more differentiated postmitotic cells (PMCs). Near the epithelial surface, the PMCs fully differentiate into terminally differentiated cells. The PMCs and the terminally differentiated cells are the suprabasal epithelial cells.[3]

Increased numbers of epithelial cells have been seen in ablated corneas. The epithelial hyperplasia is thicker at the edge of the ablation than at the center, possibly accounting for the regression of refractive error seen in patients.[8]

Pearl:
If epithelial hyperplasia is thicker at the edge of the ablation than at the center, it may account for regression.

Adhesion

The fourth and final stage, adhesion, entails the reconstruction of adhesion structures of the epithelium to Bowman's membrane.[1] The epithelium reattaches to the basement membrane and stroma with newly made hemidesmosomes and associated anchoring structures.[7] It takes 6–8 weeks for restoration of full adhesion between the epithelial cells. Before this, the adhesions are relatively weak. The cells are easily rubbed off. Hemidesmosomes, anchoring fibrils, and anchoring plaques re-establish tight adhesion to the underlying stroma.[3]

The speed of hemidesmosomal attachments depends on whether the basement membrane remains intact. In monkey eyes, if the epithelial basement membrane is fragmented, the area can be devoid of anchoring fibrils for as long as 18 months.[8] Some PRK patients experience epithelial breakdown, resulting in symptoms of foreign body sensation, lacrimation, or tenderness. Even LASIK patients can complain of recurrent foreign body sensation from recurrent erosions in the gutter. Epithelial breakdown occurs when there is a failure to establish firm anchoring points.[8]

Corneal Sensitivity and Nerve Regeneration after LASIK

Without intact nerve fibers, several key activities of wound healing are diminished. Cellular migration occurs less, epithelial mitosis decreases, and epithelial cell growth is hampered.[4] In LASIK patients, corneal hypoesthesia results, and recovery takes months after the procedure.[3] Applying a cotton wisp to test sensitivity will show hypoesthesia as the patient is followed up. The decreased sensitivity may inhibit blink rate and exacerbate any post-LASIK dryness.

Pearl:
LASIK patients have decreased corneal sensitivity for several months.

Stromal Wound Healing

The stroma undergoes its own healing process. After the wounding, keratocytes disappear when epithelial wound healing begins. This occurs within 30 minutes of the wounding.[4,5,10] Within 2 hours, keratocytes are almost completely absent in the anterior stroma.[5] In 15 hours, the cells are absent in 40% of the anterior stroma.[5,11] The keratocytes disappear by apoptosis. *Apoptosis* is the controlled death of cells, in which it is postulated that unnecessary cells are eliminated.[12] A benefit of apoptosis is minimal damage to the surrounding tissue. By minimizing collateral damage, keratocytic apoptosis helps to preserve clarity in the cornea. Another benefit of apoptosis is the closing down of any portal for infection.[10]

Keratocytes undergo proliferation and migration to regenerate the stroma after wounding. Keratocytes migrate to the surface of the wound and expand the fibroblast population by mitosis. The mitosis is not seen within the ablated zone. The repopulation occurs at the periphery of the wound, not in the wound from a migration of keratocytes from underlying basal layers of the stroma.[3] Keratocyte reproduction peaks in 3–6 days and does not begin until the new epithelium covers the corneal wound. After apoptosis, newly-activated keratocytes (fibroblasts) produce collagens, glycoproteins, and proteoglycans that form the stromal extracellular matrix.[3,10] Normal keratocytes have oval nuclei, whereas fibroblasts are spindle-shaped with dense nuclei.[13] The fibroblastic response is intense at 3 months and tapers off at 6–15 months.[3,14] Stroma has collagen types I, III, and IV, which copolymerize within the same fibrils throughout the stroma. Type VI constitutes 30% of the collagen content and is found in the connecting filaments interlinking stromal collagen fibrils.[3,4]

Newly synthesized collagen fibrils are larger in diameter and account for the haze seen after PRK. The new fibrils and extracellular matrix may also have a different index than the existing stroma.[3] Corticosteroids inhibit corneal healing and reduce deposition of scar tissue.[8,14]

Haze is drastically reduced in LASIK. Keratocyte apoptosis is thought to be the initiating event in the stromal wound healing response.[12] The apoptosis is triggered by mechanically wounding the epithelium. The epithelium releases the cytokines interleukin-1 and Fas ligand to mediate keratocyte apoptosis.[12,15,16]

With LASIK, apoptosis is undetected in the underlying stroma. However, research has shown that keratocytic loss occurs in LASIK at a reduced rate.[17] If the epithelium is intentionally damaged after LASIK, apoptosis appears in 50% or more of the anterior stroma.[12] Stromal haze is reduced when the epithelium is kept intact.

Regression is also reduced with LASIK, more so than PRK. The wound healing response is deeper in the stroma with LASIK. There is a diminished effect of activated keratocytes on the overlying epithelium. Less epithelial hypertrophy occurs, leading to less regression.[10]

Endothelial Wound Healing

There is minimal or no capacity for the eye to regenerate endothelial cells. Endothelial wound repair is generally achieved by enlarging and sliding endothelial cells. There are no short- or medium-term effects on the endothelium after LASIK.[3,18]

References

1. Abelson MB, Slugg AP. Corneal wound healing and its modulation. Rev Ophthamol 1999;November:92–105.
2. Gimbel HV, Penno EEA. Early Postoperative Complications: 24 to 48 Hours. In HV Gimbel, EEA Penno (eds), LASIK Complications. Thorofare, NJ: Slack, 1999.

3. McMenamin PG, Steele C, McGhee CNJ. Cornea: Anatomy, Physiology and Healing. In H McGhee, DS Taylor, Gartry, et al. (eds), Excimer Lasers in Ophthalmology Principle and Practice. Boston: Butterworth–Heinemann, 1997.

4. Dayhaw-Barker P. Corneal wound healing: II. The process. ICLC 1995;22:110–116.

5. Crosoon CE. Cellular Changes Following Epithelial Abrasion. In RW Beurman, CE Crosoon, HE Kaufman (eds). Healing Processes in the Cornea. Houston: Gulf Publishing, 1989.

6. Muller LJ, Pels L, Vrensen GFJM. Novel aspects of the ultrastructural organization of human corneal keratocytes. Inves Ophthalmol Vis Sci 1995;36:2557–2566.

7. Berman M. The Pathogenesis of Corneal Epithelial Defects. In RW Beurman, CE Crosoon, HE Kaufman (eds). Healing Processes in the Cornea. Houston: Gulf Publishing, 1989;15–26.

8. Tuft SJ, Gartry DS, Rawe IM, et al. Photorefractive keratectomy: implications of corneal wound healing. Br J Ophthal 1993;77:243–247.

9. Nishida T, Nakagawa S. Expression of Fibronectin Receptors in Corneal Epithelial Cells. In RW Beurman, CE Crosoon, HE Kaufman (eds), Healing Processes in the Cornea. Houston: Gulf Publishing, 1989;127–138.

10. Wilson SE. Keratocyte apoptosis: response to corneal epithelial injury. EyeWorld 1998:January;14–15.

11. Nassaralla BA, Szerenyi K, Pinheiro MN, et al. Prevention of keratocyte loss after corneal de-epithelialization in rabbits. Arch Ophthalmol 1995;113:506–511.

12. Helena MC, Baerveldt F, Kim W, et al. Keratocyte apoptosis after corneal surgery. Invest Ophthal Vis Sci 1998;39:276–283.

13. Chew S, Beurman RW, Kaufman HE, et al. In vivo confocal microscopy of corneal wound healing after excimer laser photorefractive keratectomy. CLAO J 1995;21:273–280.

14. You X, Bergmanson JPG, Zheng XM, et al. Effect of corticosteroids on rabbit corneal keratocytes after photorefractive keratectomy. J Refract Surg 1995;11:460–467.

15. Bonner H. The interaction of corneal cells and the corneal extracellular matrix. South J Optom 1998;16:12–13.

16. Snyder MC, Bergmanson JPG, Doughty MJ. Keratocytes: no more the quiet cells. J Am Optom Assoc 1998;69:180–187.

17. Autry JC, Bergmanson JPG, Sheldon TM, et al. Morphological observations of the long term corneal effects of excimer laser therapy. Optom Vis Sci 1997;74:99.

18. Kent DG, Soloman KD, Peng Q, et al. Effect of surface photorefractive keratectomy and laser in situ keratomileusis on the corneal endothelium. J Cataract Refract Surg 1997;23:386–397.

CHAPTER 3

Monovision and LASIK

Milton M. Hom

Monovision is defined as designating one eye for distance vision and the other eye for near vision.[1] Normally, monovision is performed with contact lenses. However, with the early presbyopic and midpresbyopic demographics of refractive surgery patients, monovision in LASIK is also common. Targeting one eye for distance vision and the companion eye for near vision is a common practice by many refractive surgeons.[2,3] The procedure is not commonly performed on younger, advancing myopes. Late presbyopes are not commonly chosen because of lenticular changes, which diminish monocular visual acuity. A monovision correction can ultimately be achieved during the selection of an intraocular lens implant.

Liability is a strong consideration when targeting a refractive surgery patient for monovision. The patient must be advised of the side effects and risks associated with monovision. The warnings should be documented in the patient's charts with record entries or the use of forms. Before the surgical procedure, the effect of monovision should be demonstrated through a contact lens trial.[4]

Monovision Considerations

Monovision has a reported success rate of 50–75% when performed with contact lenses.[4,5] However, the biggest drawback with monovision is night driving. A significant percentage of patients report glare during night driving.[6,7] Schor et al. report that 33% of monovision contact lens patients experience glare.[6] Josephson and Caffrey found an 80% incidence of glare with monovision or aspheric bifocals.[8] When one eye is defocused with an add, binocular distance visual acuity can be decreased. The amount of the perceived decrease in vision depends on the lighting conditions and the target size disparity. Driving at night introduces a large, out-of-focus headlight image in the near eye, and a much smaller, clearer image in the distance eye. In a high-contrast environment such as night driving, a monovision

Chapter modified from Hom MM. Monovision and LASIK. J Am Optom Assoc 1999;70:117–122.

patient displays difficulty in suppressing the out-of-focus, larger image in the near eye.[9,10] To the patient, this can be interpreted as glare.

Another disadvantage is compromised stereoacuity.[11] Stereopsis has been shown to decrease with monovision. Younger subjects 23–28 years of age have reduced stereopsis of 50 arc seconds with 2.0–2.50 D of monocular blur.[12] Although stereopsis is reduced, Koetting found 94% of his monovision patients possessed stereopsis within the norms for their age groups.[13] The range of stereopsis can vary. Lebow and Goldberg have shown a wide range of values, from no stereopsis to complete stereopsis, for monovision patients.[14]

In comparison, successful monovision patients have a much smaller reduction in stereoacuity than unsuccessful monovision patients.[15] The reduction in stereopsis is probably related to the strength of interocular blur suppression (see the section Interocular Blur Suppression). Patients with stronger interocular blur suppression make better monovision patients.[10] Despite the compromised stereoacuity, peripheral visual acuity remains largely unaffected.[16] The compromise is limited to central vision. There seems to be some adaptation to monovision.[17] Despite the initial reduction in stereopsis, stereoacuity has been shown to increase after 3 weeks of monovision.

It has been argued that stereopsis is relatively unimportant for driving. Under dynamic conditions, the contribution of stereopsis is minimal for distances over 20 feet. Other monocular clues are more important for depth perception while driving. The relative motion of the visual field provides monocular clues for depth perception. Perspective, speed of motion, overlapping contours, and dynamically changing disparities are all contributing factors to monocular clues.[7]

Interocular Blur Suppression

The ability of the brain and the eye to suppress detrimental blurred information from the near eye during distance viewing has been referred to as *interocular blur suppression.*[9,10] Interocular blur suppression aids distance binocular vision. With the suppression mechanism in place, only a small reduction in distance acuity occurs with monovision.

Interocular blur suppression enables monovision to work. If interocular blur suppression is not present, a mixture of blurred and clear vision at all distances results. Under dim light conditions, the binocular suppression of blur becomes less effective. This accounts for the poor visual performance of monovision in activities such as night driving.[10]

The strength of interocular blur suppression affects the success of potential monovision patients. Successful monovision patients have interocular suppression of blur 100 times greater than that of unsuccessful patients.[10]

Interocular blur suppression is usually not complete. The information from the blurred portions of the image continues to be processed with the in-focus image. Although the highly detailed portions of the defocused eye cannot be used, the larger features (medium- and low-frequency components) are processed. The brain uses retinal image disparity of the larger features to allow partial or reduced stereopsis.[10]

Monovision Trial

Most clinicians agree the best way to demonstrate the effects of monovision preoperatively is a monovision trial with contact lenses.[18,19] A monovision trial can be performed with spectacles; however, due to the differences in relative spectacle magnification between glasses and contact lenses, a contact lens trial more accurately simulates vision after the procedure. Spectacle monovision induces unwanted magnification or minification effects. The peripheral vision may also be inhibited by surrounding frames, eyewire, and aberrations.

Unless significant astigmatism is present, soft contact lenses are most convenient for a contact lens trial. Sample disposable lenses or planned replacement lenses can be used. The trial is normally 1–2 weeks, but can take up to 6 weeks.[7] Daily disposable lenses may also be used, giving the added advantage of no disinfection needed. Other lenses, such as rigid gas-permeable lenses (RGPs), may be used but do not have the disposability of soft lenses. Longer adaptation times for an RGP wearer are normally required, and a longer de-adaptation is required to achieve pre-fitting refractive and keratometric stability before the procedure. Despite the disadvantages of RGPs, the afforded visual quality is usually better than that of soft lenses.

Distance Eye and Near Eye

There are different philosophies regarding the designation of which eye is preferred for distance vision and which eye for near vision. Sometimes refractive error is used as a guideline.[20] Eye dominance can be used as a selection criterion. Normally, the nondominant eye is used for near and the dominant eye for distance. However, studies have shown that choosing the dominant eye for distance does not necessarily produce the better vision.

Despite these facts, use of the dominant sighting eye for distance may still be the best strategy. Keep in mind, however, that some patients do not have a sighting preference.[20] Asking the patient questions such as "Which eye do you use for a telescope/microscope/camera?" or "Which eye do you use for sighting when shooting?" can give the answers to which eye is dominant.

The *anisometropic blur test* identifies a higher percentage of these patients than other methods of determining eye dominance. Anisometropic blur test compares the contrast necessary to see a target clearly. An aperture subtending a visual angle of 12 minutes of arc is back illuminated with a 60-W bulb. Background luminance is controlled by a bulb providing front illumination. Subjects wear a monovision set-up in contact lenses. The target first appears blurred under high contrast. The rheostat on the front bulb is then adjusted to increase background luminance (and decrease contrast) until the target is perceived as clear. The procedure is then repeated with the near lens over the opposite eye. The sensory dominant eye is the one needing the lowest background luminance (and the highest contrast) to see clearly.[21]

The dominant eye is superior for spatial-locomotor tasks, such as walking, running, and driving a car. The nondominant eye may also be better suited for near tasks. Tasks such as reading do not require a precise sense of absolute visual direction.[10]

Dominance can also be determined by having the patient form a gap between the thumb and forefinger of the two hands. While extending his or her arms, the patient sights a distant target through the gap. The eye used to sight the target is chosen as the distance eye.

The *swinging-plus test* can be used to select the near eye. The patient walks around the room with a +1.50 D lens over one eye. The test is repeated with the lens over the other eye. The most comfortable eye with the plus lens becomes the near eye.[22]

Another test to help determine dominance is *near point of convergence*. The eye that loses fixation first can be chosen as the distance eye. The eye that continues to fixate on the target as it approaches is the choice for the near eye.

Sometimes handedness is used to determine dominance. For example, if the patient is right-handed, some practitioners would designate the right eye for distance.

In some cases, the same eye can be dominant for both distance and near tasks. Switching the eye function during the trial period may be necessary.

Selection of Add Power

There are two conflicting philosophies when choosing an add power. One philosophy is to pick the smallest power possible. The smallest power helps to maximize binocular function. Preservation of binocular summation, better stereopsis, and more stable interocular suppression are advantages of lower add powers. The other philosophy is choosing the maximum power tolerated by the patient. Higher add powers help to stabilize the blur suppression needed for monovision to work.[23]

When patients are presented with dissimilar contours, such as vectographic targets, suppression is enhanced with higher adds.[23] Schor et al., however, have shown that interocular blur suppression becomes less stable with higher adds.[10] For the best visual performance with monovision, binocular summation should be maximized.

Binocular Summation

When two eyes are used instead of one, visual performance greatly increases. This is called *binocular summation*. The binocular contrast sensitivity is approximately 42% higher than monocular contrast sensitivity. When the visual performance is worse binocularly than monocularly, it is called *binocular inhibition*. Pardhan and Gilchrist have shown that monovision adds up to +1.50 D produce binocular summation.[15] Adds higher than +1.50 D produce binocular inhibition.[15,24] To best take advantage of binocular summation, adds less than +1.50 D should be prescribed.

A closer look at the study by Pardhan and Gilchrist[15] shows that the critical add power when binocular summation crosses over to binocular inhibition is between +1.00 and +1.50 D. We have found clinically the best add power to target for our early LASIK presbyopes is +1.25 to +1.50 D, the maximum add affording the patient binocular summation.

For older presbyopes, we use a +1.50 D add. However, as shown by Lebow and Goldberg, add powers in monovision can range greatly between +0.37 and +2.75 D.[14] The add power should ultimately be determined by the monovision contact lens trial (see below). One interesting note is that Lebow and Goldberg's average add power was +1.50 D. Patients with add powers less than +1.25 D will generally meet the minimum visual acuity requirements for driving with either eye.[7] Another rule of thumb for choosing add power for monovision contact lenses is the *rule of two-thirds*. Giving the patient two-thirds of the add power provides enhanced acuity without introducing binocular problems.[25] For an early presbyope requiring a +1.00 D add, targeting a +0.62 D add is common.

Age is another consideration when selecting add powers for patients in their late 30s. For patients not yet old enough to be presbyopic (e.g., 38 years of age), undercorrection of one eye should be considered. Although the patient does not need the add power, monovision can be targeted for future benefit. Many patients close to presbyopia take advantage of monovision earlier than needed. However, if the patient does not have near blur with their distance correction, it is difficult for him or her to accept a blurry eye postoperatively. Again, the monovision trial should be the determining test.

If the patient has a refractive error around –1.00 to –2.50 D, a monovision surgical trial can be performed. Instead of a bilateral procedure, just one eye can be targeted for Plano. The other eye is left alone and used as the near eye. If the patient is unable to adapt, the other eye can be targeted for Plano, taking away the monovision.

Initial Fitting

During the initial trial contact lens monovision fitting, the patient should be given the opportunity to wear the lenses in the office. Patients should be encouraged to negotiate up and down stairs and perform distance- and near-vision tasks. If the patient experiences an adverse reaction or poor response, monovision may not be a good choice for the patient. Patients prone to motion sickness may be at higher risk for a poor response. If the patient shows good adaptability with minor difficulties, there is an excellent chance of success.[18]

Management

Continued follow-up for monovision should take place over several weeks for adaptation. The capability to make changes for better adaptation before surgery is a major benefit of a contact lens trial. Normal symptoms of adaptation are hazy vision, eye strain, and mild eye switching.[26] As mentioned previously, sometimes switching the distance and near eyes can relieve even the mildest of symptoms. The distance eye becomes the near eye and vice versa.[27]

Because of the night-driving difficulties previously discussed, it may be advisable for the patient to wear the monovision trial lenses first as a passenger before attempting to drive. Patients with little visual compromise can ease into driving by initially limiting themselves to short distances and daylight hours.[26] One of the major purposes of the monovision trial is to gain experience with night driving.

If there are difficulties with the contact lenses, common fitting problems should be ruled out first. These problems include residual cylinder, incorrect powers, and poor fit. In some cases, soft toric lenses may be indicated for the monovision trial.

Residual astigmatism can play a major role in problematic distance vision. A spherical cylinder over-refraction is highly recommended to detect even the smallest amounts of uncorrected astigmatism. Residual astigmatism of –1.00 DC has been shown to induce a significant two-line reduction in distance acuity for monovision. If the residual astigmatism is at an oblique axis, a further reduction of one to two letters can be expected. Correcting amounts smaller than –1.00 may prove worthwhile to achieve optimal distance acuity.[9] The lowest amount a toric soft lens can presently correct is –0.50 DC. Nonetheless, a sphero-cylindrical cylinder over-refraction is indicated for monovision patients.

Intermediate blur is a common complaint about monovision. Adding minus to the near eye can relieve this symptom. However, by adding minus, the near vision will be compromised. Adding plus to the distance eye is another strategy to consider.[1] However, concomitantly with adding plus, distance vision can be compromised. Keep in mind that small 0.25 D changes can make a large difference when adjusting the power for monovision patients.

Spectacle Overcorrection

Sometimes a spectacle overcorrection is needed after the procedure. For night driving or reading small print, a compensatory spectacle can give the patient the added clear vision to be comfortable.[7] For a patient using the right eye for distance and the left eye for near, an example of this correction would be RE Plano LE –1.50 DS. Monovision is considered successful if it is satisfactory 80% of the time and spectacles over monovision are needed for only 15–20% of the time.[1] If monovision is unsatisfactory, an enhancement can return both eyes to binocular vision.

Gradual Transitioning

A monovision trial with contact lenses may not portray adaptation to patients. The contact lens trial will demonstrate monovision in a spontaneous manner. Due to regression, a LASIK patient will gradually transition into monovision. For instance, in the author's experience, a typical patient will be +0.75 D in the distance eye and Plano in the near eye 1 week after surgery. After a period of 3–4 weeks, the eyes should regress to Plano in the distance eye and –0.75 D in the near eye. Because the regression occurs over a period of 3–4 weeks, the patient has an extended and gradual transition into monovision. A contact lens trial, however, is not gradual. The trial is an almost instantaneous step into monovision. Therefore, an unsuccessful contact lens trial does not necessarily mean an unsuccessful monovision LASIK patient.

Advancing Presbyopia

Because of the need for increasing adds as the patient ages, the usefulness of monovision may diminish with time. The patient should understand that his or her ability to read will likely change in the future. The need for more plus power at near can be treated with a spectacle over the monovision. For a year or so after the procedure, wearing the spectacles only 15% of the time may be considered a success. However, as the years pass, that percentage will only increase.

References

1. Hom MM. Monovision and Bifocals. In MM Hom (ed), Manual of Contact Lens Prescribing and Fitting. Boston: Butterworth–Heinemann, 1997:327–354.
2. Beran RF, Doty J. Laser Assisted In Situ Keratomileusis (LASIK). In RF Beran, Doty J (eds), The Surgical Management of Myopia and Astigmatism: A Guide for Optometrists. Columbus, OH: Anadem Publishing, 1996:87–101.

 3. Lingua RW (ed). The Essentials of LASIK and Its Comanagement. Brea, CA: TLC Laser Center, 1997.
 4. Gauthier CA, Holden BA, Grant T, et al. Interest of presbyopes in contact lens correction and their success with monovision. Optom Vis Sci 1992;69:858–862.
 5. Shapiro MB, Bredson DC. Premarket evaluation of Unilens RGP aspheric multifocal contact lens. CL Spectrum 1992;7:21–24.
 6. Schor CM, Carson M, Peterson G, et al. Effects of interocular blur suppression ability on monovision tasks performance. JAOA 1989;60:188–192.
 7. Josephson JE, Erickson P, Back A. Monovision. JAOA 1990;61:820–826.
 8. Josephson JE, Caffrey BE. Monovision vs. bifocal contact lenses. A crossover study. JAOA 1987;58:652–654.
 9. Collins M, Goode A, Brown B. Distance visual acuity and monovision. Optom Vis Sci 1993;70:723–728.
10. Schor C, Landsman L, Erickson P. Ocular dominance and the interocular suppression of blur in monovision. Am J Optom Physiol Opt 1987;64:723–730.
11. Back A, Grant T, Hine N. Comparative visual performance of three presbyopic contact lens corrections. Optom Vis Sci 1992;69:474–480.
12. Jain S, Arora I, Azar DT. Monovision Refractive Surgery. In DT Azar (ed), Refractive Surgery. Stamford, CT: Appleton and Lange, 1997:135–142.
13. Koetting RA. Stereopsis and presbyopes fitted with single vision contact lenses. Am J Optom Arch Am Acad Optom 1970;47:557–561.
14. Lebow KA, Goldberg JB. Characteristics of binocular vision found for presbyopic patients wearing single vision contact lenses. JAOA 1975;46:1116–1123.
15. Pardhan S, Gilchrist J. The effect of monocular defocus on binocular contrast sensitivity. Ophthal Physio Opt 1990;10:33–36.
16. Collins MJ, Brown B, Verney S, et al. Peripheral visual acuity with monovision and other contact lens corrections for presbyopia. Optom Vis Sci 1989;66:370–374.
17. Harris MG. Sheedy JE, Gan CM. Vision and task performance with monovision and diffractive bifocal contact lenses. Optom Vis Sci 1992;69:609–614.
18. Harris MG, Classe JG. Clinicolegal considerations of monovision. JAOA 1988;59:491–495.
19. Maguen E, Nesburn AB, Salz JJ. Bilateral photokeratorefractive keratectomy with intentional unilateral undercorrection in an aircraft pilot. J Cataract Refract Surg 1997;23:294–296.
20. Jain S, Arora I, Azar DT. Success of monovision in presbyopes: review of the literature and potential applications to refractive surgery. Surv Ophthal 1996;40:491–499.
21. Robboy MW, Cox IG, Erickson P. Effects of sighting and sensory dominance on monovision high and low contrast visual acuity. CLAO J 1990;16:299–301.
22. Stein HA. The management of presbyopia with contact lenses: a review. CLAO J 1990;16:33–38.
23. Heath DA, Hines C, Schwartz F. Suppression behavior analyzed as a function of monovision addition power. Optom Vis Sci 1986;63:198–201.

24. Loshin DS, Loshin MS, Comer G. Binocular summation with monovision contact lens correction for presbyopia. ICLC 1982;9:161–165.
25. Rigel L. Which modality works best? When monovision makes sense. Rev Opt 1998;135:90.
26. Harris MG, Classe JG. Clinicolegal considerations of monovision. JAOA 1988;59:491–495.
27. Bennett ES, Henry VA. Bifocal Contact Lenses. In ES Bennett, VA Henry (eds), Clinical Manual of Contact Lenses. Philadelphia: Lippincott, 1994:362–398.

CHAPTER 4

Preprocedure Selection and Workup

Charlotte Burns

Primary eye care practitioners are in the unique position to introduce and co-manage qualified patients to refractive laser surgery. This position enables the primary eye care practitioner to be in the front line of educating prospective patients. The material addresses the process of educating patients and prospective candidates in two parts. The first portion offers practical advice to the practitioner who seeks to introduce the concept of refractive laser surgery to patient candidates. The latter portion helps to inform the primary eye care practitioner of the technical aspects of deciding whether a patient is a more appropriate candidate for photorefractive keratectomy (PRK) or LASIK.

The preoperative patient evaluation and workup is an important factor in predicting a patient's satisfaction with laser vision correction. Counseling before the surgery has a significant impact on the patient's expectations and influences his or her feelings about whether to consider the surgery a success or failure.

Many patients consider refractive surgery an attractive alternative to corrective lenses, and with time, the number of patient inquiries will greatly increase. The vast majority of patients considering laser vision correction require an extended educational process. It is not unusual for a patient to wait several months after their initial consultation before proceeding with refractive surgery.

Pearl:
It is not unusual for patients to wait several months after their initial consultation to have LASIK.

Laser vision correction should be reviewed as an option for patients in the same manner as contact lenses or glasses. It can be part of the examination routine to introduce the topic to potential candidates. Many complications are avoidable with proper follow-up. The patient will benefit from the follow-up that optometric co-management has to offer.

Consultative Process

The consultative process for refractive surgery should include the risks, benefits, limitations, and reasonable expectations of the procedure. Proper patient management requires that the practitioner discuss patient expectations and fulfill medical-legal responsibilities. A conservative approach has proved the most effective. It is best to discuss the different types of refractive surgery options and to explain the benefits and risks associated with each. LASIK may offer candidates the ability to correct a high degree of myopia with rapid visual rehabilitation; however, there is greater risk intraoperatively than with other procedures such as PRK. LASIK has the greater refractive predictability associated with photoablation, but without significant risk of subepithelial haze formation. The newer refractive procedures, such as intracorneal ring segments and phakic intraocular lenses, may offer better vision, but they have their respective disadvantages (see Chapter 11, Future Techniques and Investigational Procedures).

All options of vision correction (glasses, contact lenses, and laser vision correction) should be presented to patients to assist in their understanding of the manner in which the corrective measure improves their vision. When the LASIK and PRK procedures are explained to the patient, the patient can be told that both procedures are designed to change the curvature of the eye to match that of their prescription, contact lenses, or glasses. It is then incumbent to explain the differences in the procedures and to explain the risk-benefit analysis of each procedure as it applies to the patient's condition.

An example of a patient-oriented discussion follows: The laser changes the curvature of the cornea, whether on the surface of the eye or in the deeper layers of the cornea. The surface of the eye is more reactive and sensitive, requiring a longer healing time and more eye drops. Therefore, when a procedure requires a great amount of tissue removal to correct moderate or high myopia, it is preferable to treat the deeper layers with LASIK rather than superficially with PRK. PRK's predictability has been extremely high for low degrees of myopia, and the risk of serious complications extremely low. However, some surgeons prefer LASIK over PRK for even low myopes because of superior healing.[1,2]

PRK is associated with a greater risk of infection, 1/1,000 compared to 1/5,000 with LASIK. PRK is also associated with more pain, 1/10 versus 1/50 with LASIK. The risk of scarring or haze after PRK is 1% or less with low degrees of correction, but as high as 5% for higher degrees. The risk of haze with LASIK is less than 0.2% for all degrees of correction.[1]

Visual recovery for PRK is slower, 1–2 weeks, compared to 1–7 days with LASIK. Steroid medications are needed for PRK for months. If the surgeon chooses to prescribe steroids after LASIK, the course is usually 1 week or less (see Chapter 7, Postprocedure Management). Keep in mind that there are attendant risks with the long-term use of steroids (Table 4.1).

TABLE 4.1
Comparison of Photorefractive Keratectomy and LASIK

Side Effects	Photorefractive Keratectomy	Laser In Situ Keratomileusis (LASIK)
Infection	1/1,000–1/3,500	1/50
Pain	1/10	1/50
Night glare	2%	2%
Loss of best-corrected visual acuity	1%	1%
Scarring/healing haze	1–5%	0.1%
Corneal flap risks	N/A	1/500 (depending on skill level of surgeon)
Undercorrection	Varies with prescription	Varies with prescription
Overcorrection	1%	1%
Steroid drops	1–6 mos	4–7 days
Visual recovery	1–2 wks	1–7 days

Source: Modified from JJ Machat (ed). Excimer Laser Refractive Surgery: Practice and Principles. Thorofare, NJ: Slack, 1996.

The main disadvantage with LASIK is that a cut is involved, which adds the risk of a serious complication. Flap complications include, but are not limited to, the following: a buttonhole, a partial flap, or a corneal perforation[2,3] (see Chapter 8, LASIK Complications and Management). A nontechnical way to explain the LASIK procedure and instrumentation is to describe the microkeratome as a very small carpenter's plane used to create a corneal flap.

Because corneal tissue is ablated, corneal thickness can be an issue for higher myopes (see Chapter 6, Description of Primary Procedure and Retreatment). This can be a problem for patients with more than –6.00 D of myopia, and it is good to prepare such patients for the possibility that all their myopia may not be corrected. It is appropriate to say that LASIK is considered to be the best procedure, but that all procedures must be considered in terms of their risk to benefit ratio for each patient. It is always safer to treat one eye at a time; however, most patients, especially higher myopes, prefer to have simultaneous bilateral surgery. Bilateral surgery with

LASIK may be safer than with PRK, because 95% of the complications with LASIK occur intraoperatively, compared to the 95% of PRK complications that occur postoperatively.

Pearl:
Ninety-five percent of LASIK complications occur intraoperatively, whereas 95% of PRK complications occur postoperatively.

The most important factors to many patients contemplating LASIK are the speed of recovery and the low amount of pain involved. Most people desire a procedure that disrupts their life as little as possible, and most find it difficult to proceed with any procedure that produces pain even with significant long-term value.

As with all refractive procedures, the goal of laser vision correction is to reduce the functional dependence of the patient on corrective lenses. It cannot be guaranteed that the procedure will completely eliminate the need for corrective lenses. The fact that a laser is used appears to build unrealistic patient expectations; therefore, it is important to stress the fact that patients may not be completely free of correction. A large part of surgical success for a patient depends on their individual healing.

Pearl:
Sometimes the use of a laser builds unrealistic expectations in the patient.

The consultative process is aimed at dealing with two fundamental elements: patient expectations and surgical complications. The latter is important from a medical-legal perspective, but the former is essential to produce satisfied patients. Patients must understand that even good candidates may still require glasses for certain activities such as reading or night driving. Success is defined as meeting patient expectations rather than a visual goal.

In the consultation process, patients typically pose four central concerns:

1. What is the best result I can achieve?
2. What is the worst possible outcome?
3. What are the costs involved?
4. What are the surgeon's qualifications?

What Is the Best Result the Patient Can Hope For?

The best manner to address the question "What is the best result the patient can hope for?" is to base the answer in terms of statistical success rates achieving a given level of visual acuity. There is often a perceived discrepancy, however, between what is considered a successful outcome and what is satisfactory to many individuals. Success rates are generally based on achieving legal driving vision of 20/40 uncorrected visual acuity. However, most patients and practitioners consider 20/25 uncorrected visual acuity or better as successful.

The patient who has worn rigid gas-permeable lenses, and has experienced 20/15 visual acuity with those lenses, may have a difficult time adjusting to even 20/20 uncorrected visual acuity postoperatively. It seems patients with 0.75 D or more of residual myopia still desire further correction, regardless of the severity of their preoperative refractive error.

It has proved advantageous to demonstrate 20/40 vision to patients to help them develop reasonable expectations. Otherwise, patients will compare their final acuity post–laser vision correction to their best corrected acuity before the procedure, and the surgical result falls short of their expectations. It is important to discuss anything that may leave vision at a suboptimal level, such as monovision. It is a good idea to help them experience monovision either with contact lenses, spectacle lenses, or through the phoropter[4] (see Chapter 3, Monovision and LASIK).

A problem that patients may encounter postoperatively is that, instead of recognition of the great quantitative improvement achieved, they experience qualitative vision loss. In other words, patients may achieve 20/20 visual acuity yet be unsatisfied because of loss of qualitative vision. For example, the patient may experience central islands or small optical zones producing night glare. This is a difficult concept for a patient to comprehend preoperatively.

Experience in interviewing postoperative patients indicates that even a satisfied patient will comment on some aspect of his or her vision that the patient does not regard as optimal. Neither Snellen acuity or contrast sensitivity can adequately give an idea of complete optical performance, and optical performance will likely be diminished in some manner in most patients. However, only a very small percentage of these people will be severely affected by that reduction. Patient expectations and complications are intertwined with the optical performance issue and should be explained in advance of surgery.

What Is the Worst Possible Outcome?

It is apparent to all that the worst possible outcome is blindness. All patients considering refractive surgery are fearful of losing their eyesight, which is why many patients, regardless of how motivated they are, will never proceed with any refractive surgery. The potential for laser vision correction to produce irreversible harm to an eye should not be overlooked, as there are reported cases of legal blindness with PRK and LASIK. Some surgeons even discuss possible death, which could occur secondary to cardiac arrhythmias.

Death and blindness are within the realm of possibility, however, the loss of best corrected acuity is most likely the worst outcome experienced. Patients have difficulty comprehending what this actually means. The best way to explain a loss of best corrected vision is to explain that it generally involves a loss of sharpness, crispness, or clarity of vision that glasses or contact lenses cannot restore. The loss is similar in nature to wearing glasses that are a few years out of date. It can also be helpful to show the patient through the phoropter 2–3 lines less than their best corrected acuity, to help prepare them for a less than optimal outcome.

Pearl:
Showing the patient 2–3 lines less than their best corrected visual acuity can help prepare them for a less than optimal outcome.

It is important to alert patients that most patients experience a loss of qualitative vision immediately after surgery. Most people improve within 2–4 weeks, 99% percent improve over 6 months, and a small percentage, 1%, will never improve. There can be a sense of panic after surgery if vision is not perfectly clear. The patient may believe that something went wrong with his or her surgery. If informed before surgery, the patient is aware that vision may have a degree of blurriness immediately after, that this is normal, and that it may require months to improve.

Pearl:
Most patients experience loss of qualitative vision immediately following the procedure.

Night glare is another important side effect to address, as it is almost a certain immediate postoperative experience. This will clear gradually over months in most patients and is optical zone dependent. It is a good idea to document pupil size before surgery and at each postoperative visit. If the patient has large pupils, it would be prudent to warn the patient of the higher risk of night glare and have this documented in his or her chart.

What Are the Financial Costs Involved?

Financial cost is an issue that must be addressed appropriately; the financial obligations are a significant consideration for many patients. Co-management fees should be disclosed to the patient. A variety of financing options can be made available. Any patients who base their decision to proceed with refractive surgery on the savings of never having to purchase corrective lenses again should be dissuaded from proceeding with any refractive procedure. The reality is that they may require corrective lenses of some type after surgery.

If patients recognize and perceive that the procedure will add value to their quality of life, the majority do not find the costs prohibitive. When the excimer laser was first approved in the United States, many doctors believed that the only patients who would be willing to undergo the procedure would be wealthy patients. However, a high percentage of patients who have undergone laser vision correction do not have a great deal of disposable income. There are, and always will be, individuals who seek out the least costly vision correction modality or refractive center, regardless of any other consideration.

What Are the Qualifications of the Surgeon?

Complications are an inherent part of any surgical procedure. A surgeon who says he or she never has a complication is one who never performs surgery. With more surgeons performing LASIK, many are courting optometric referrals. As with all patient referral and co-management, it is important to keep the patient's well-being in mind.

Patient Education

Visual complications are especially traumatic, as the patient lives with a poor outcome during every waking hour. It is because humans are so visual that refractive surgery has the ability to dramatically improve the quality of a patient's life. Conversely, complications can be just as detrimental to that quality of life (Figure 4.1). There are now cases of legal blindness that have been reported for LASIK; therefore, the potential for LASIK to produce real and irreversible harm to the eye cannot be overstated.

Refractive surgery, although a life-changing event for many people, is not for everyone. It is a viable option for a defined group of individuals within the population. The potential market varies with many factors, such as cost and availability. Risks acceptable to one person may not be acceptable to another. Each must define his or her own parameters of acceptability.

When first dealing with refractive surgery candidates, many doctors believe they have some level of responsibility for the outcome and the patient's decision to proceed. It is essential to know how to counsel the patient; however, the decision to proceed is solely the patient's choice. The doctor should only offer an unbiased presentation of information for the patient to accept or decline.

The referring doctor should ensure that the patient is well-informed. For example, the following statement may be used: "From what I understand, you are a good candidate and I would expect you to do well, but the decision to proceed is yours. I will be happy to care for you after the surgery if you decide to proceed." The surgeon should also go to great lengths to

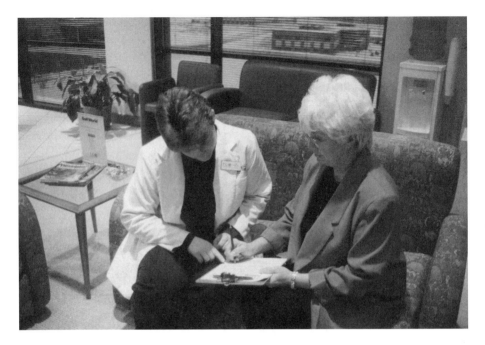

FIGURE 4.1. Patient signing the informed consent.

ensure the patient is well-informed, but should never guarantee results. The surgeon's guarantee should be limited solely to his or her best efforts.

Usually, an informed consent is not required to be signed in the co-managing doctor's office, but many doctors prefer to have that extra assurance of the patient's understanding. However, some co-managing practitioners believe that signing the informed consent in their offices is an absolute necessity. The following are recommendations for informed consent, whether in the co-managing doctor's office or the surgeon's office (note: the first three recommendations are not commonly practiced):

- The patient should write in his or her own handwriting the personal motivation for surgery.
- The patient should write in his or her own handwriting the possible need for corrective eyewear despite surgery.
- The patient should write in his or her own handwriting the significant risks of surgery.
- The patient should appreciate the risks of unilateral versus bilateral simultaneous surgery.
- There should be an avoidance of any form of implicit or explicit guarantees.

- There should be an avoidance of any advertising stating that the procedure is safe without qualifying such a statement.
- There should be an avoidance of any advertising specifying throwing away glasses or implying permanent freedom from corrective eyewear.
- The patient should not sign the consent form when dilated or under the influence of any medication not normally taken.
- The surgeon should be part of the informed consent process and meet with the patient to review risks personally before surgery.
- The patient should also be informed, usually by the surgeon, about alternative techniques and future technology.

The preoperative evaluation is based on patient education by the entire staff. Many patients are simply seeking information when they inquire or schedule a consultation. A good philosophy to maintain is that more information is better than less information. The benefits are easy for the patient to understand, and the risks are important for the patient to understand and accept. Many candidates are actually less likely to consent to the procedure if he or she does not have a full understanding of the risks. In this case, negatives add credibility to positives. When fully educating the patient, you eliminate the fear of the unknown. This must be done preoperatively. Good communication also results in happier patients.

The success rate for good candidates with lower prescriptions (–6.00 D or less and/or less than 3.00 D of astigmatism) is between 90% and 99% for 20/40 or better vision. However, only approximately 75% achieve 20/25 or better vision.[1] Therefore, it is best to describe the outcome in terms of specific activities rather than an achieved level of visual acuity, such as vision that is good enough to play sports, watch television, and drive a car without correction. For most people, the vision that is achieved is good enough to be functionally independent of glasses for 85% of activities requiring good distance vision, but glasses for reading, night driving, or bad weather driving may be required.

Success

Success, goals, and limitations of the procedure must be defined in the preoperative consultative process. A patient must understand that 20/20 acuity alone does not define success. Achieving the best vision possible in the safest, most conservative manner is the goal.

Patients must understand that the laser will not transform their eyes into emmetropic eyes, but will simply be transforming myopic eyes into eyes that have a reduced dependence on glasses. The need for continued annual dilated retinal examinations is critical, especially in higher myopes, and should be addressed. Many patients have the misconception that their risk of retinal tears and retinal detachments will be reduced. They do not understand the differences between the structures of the eye, and sometimes believe their retinal potential will improve simply because they appear to no longer be myopic. If a patient has reduced best corrected acuity before the procedure, the patient needs to understand, and it should be documented that the patient understands, their retinal potential is not likely to improve.

Pearl:
It is a misconception that LASIK reduces the risk of retinal tears and detachments. Dilated retinal examinations are still necessary.

In counseling patients, one must be careful about making misleading statements about the possible outcomes. The Federal Trade Commission has addressed advertising for laser refractive procedures. Making statements such as "The procedure is permanent and safe without long-term complications" is unwise, as these facts have yet to be determined in absolute terms. "You will be able to throw away your glasses" is also a poor and often incorrect statement.

It is reasonable to state what is known about laser vision correction results and to give personal opinions to address patient concerns (i.e., "From everything we know to date, the procedure appears to be safe"; "The LASIK procedure was first performed in 1990 and the results appear to remain stable after the first 6–12 months"; "The procedure has been performed thousands of times around the world in over 50 countries"). In reality, the risk of a serious, sight-threatening complication is less than 1%. At this point, the excimer laser has been in use for PRK for 13 years, with LASIK having been in use for 10 years. Long-term effects beyond that are unknown; however, the opinion is based on our understanding of the mechanism by which the laser works to improve vision. Thus, in a few more years, the long-term effects will not be known much beyond what is known today. The limited removal of tissue, the lack of thermal collateral damage, the retained corneal stability, and the safety of the endothelium provide ample evidence for long-term safety.

Consultative Review of Patient Risks

Eye care practitioners need to recognize that patients are overwhelmed by the entire consultative process, and that they will forget many of the complications and expectations raised and explained during their examination. When reviewing the risks it is important to first state, "These are the risks of the procedure," and to enumerate the risks in lay terms, clearly and precisely. Documentation is as important as the discussion itself. Having an assistant taking notes during the discussion is advisable.

Infection is probably the simplest risk for patients to understand, and the risk for a serious infection with LASIK is 1 in 5,000. The risk of infection for PRK is 1 in 1,000 to 1 in 3,500. Lid hygiene and broad spectrum antibiotic prophylaxis can reduce the incidence by 50%. The greatest risk is during the first few postoperative days; therefore, patients are given antibiotic medication before and after surgery as prophylaxis.

Pain should not be experienced during the procedure itself. Postoperative pain usually starts 30–90 minutes after surgery and is extremely variable. Medications are typically given to help patients sleep and avoid any discomfort. Pain is usually only a problem the first 12–24 hours for a patient without a complication, due to the epithelial defect.[5] Although reports are anecdotal, it seems that female patients tolerate these procedures better than male patients.

Patients can be light sensitive for this period of time, and it is important for them to have ultraviolet protection for the first 6 months after surgery, as ultraviolet light has been shown to cause regression in post-laser patients with LASIK.[6] Vision can be poor for the first 12 hours, improving drastically by 24 hours. The quantitative improvement during the first 24 hours is impressive; over the next month, vision improves a fraction of the original 24 hours. PRK is a little slower. The epithelial defect typically heals in 18–72 hours, with quantitative improvement over the next few days.

Regression

Regression may be a problem in a small number of patients, especially those with severe myopia preoperatively. Therefore, the success rate is lower for these patients, and simply decreased myopia may be the achieved outcome. Contacts are well tolerated after surgery, and soft lenses may be fit one week after surgery if needed. Enhancements for LASIK are performed when the patient's refraction becomes stable. The flap is most easily lifted in the first 3–6 months; however, there have been accounts of flaps being lifted after 7 years. Generally, after 6 months some surgeons will cut a flap instead of lifting the original. PRK enhancements should also be delayed until the refraction is stable and should take place at least 1 month after discontinuing steroid drops. Most centers do not charge for enhancements for a period of time, typically 1–2 years. However, some centers have no enhancement grace period. An unsatisfied patient who must pay additional fees for an enhancement is much more likely to be litigious.

Night Glare

Night glare was a problem with RK and with excimer laser PRK using smaller ablation zones. Some studies have shown that LASIK using single zone ablation actually yields a larger effective optical zone than PRK, and may have decreased glare. Patients who experience night glare tend to improve with time and once both eyes have had surgery. Patients at greatest risk remain those with large pupils and moderate to severe myopia. Additionally, patients with night glare preoperatively will usually have night glare postoperatively.

Healing Haze

Healing haze is due to collagen protein produced in the cornea during the remodeling of the eye. It is almost never visible to the naked eye, only microscopically, and generally does not produce a fog or a blur for the patient. It usually develops 1–2 weeks after LASIK. The incidence of haze with LASIK is 1 in 1,000 (0.1%). The incidence of haze with PRK is 1% below –6.00 D, but rises up to 5% above –6.00, and 3 D of cylinder. Sometimes a short steroid regimen may improve the clinical appearance, but the haze typically disappears on its own over the course of a year.

Overcorrections

Overcorrections failing to regress are likely the most troublesome and difficult patient management problem. Depending on the nomogram and excimer laser system used, this usually occurs in 2%–3% of patients. Initial overcorrection is sometimes planned, as a certain amount of regression is expected.[6] Higher prescriptions tend to be much more hyperopic immediately following surgery. Patients need reassurance during this time, as reading will be difficult for a few weeks for all patients except ones with an undercorrection. Hyperopic LASIK is now available in the United States to help treat overcorrections.

Undercorrection

The undercorrection rate varies according to the prescription. The higher the prescription, the more likely the patient will be undercorrected. If needed, the enhancement for LASIK is generally performed at least three months after surgery to ensure corneal stability.

Loss of Best Corrected Visual Acuity

Loss of best corrected visual acuity remains the most significant complication observed. Incidence varies with technique, laser system, and degree of preoperative myopia. Patients need to understand this concept, as it occurs in 1% of patients. A good way to demonstrate this concept is to show them a line around 20/40 or higher, and let them know they may not be able to read that line after surgery, even with glasses or soft contact lenses.

Flap Complications

Flap complications include thin and perforated corneal flaps, buttonhole flaps, free caps, pupil bisection, and perforated corneas.[2] After surgery, there is always the possibility of the patient's rubbing his or her eye or blinking and displacing the flap. The most critical time for this to occur is within 48 hours after surgery. After 48 hours, it generally requires significant trauma to the eye to move the flap. Great care should be taken at the surgery center, and by the co-managing doctor, to educate the patient about the importance of keeping hands away from the eyes at this time.

The flap may be lifted and floated to replace, but it is often difficult to remove the wrinkles that have formed, and often the best corrected acuity is reduced. Time is of the essence: The faster striae are resolved, the better the visual outcome.

Presbyopia

Presbyopia must be carefully explained to each candidate, but special care must be taken with the prepresbyopic group. Patients who participate in sports and social activities, drive, and watch television will benefit from binocular distance vision; however, avid readers and individuals who perform near work during the workday must balance any benefits achieved with clear distance vision against the future need for reading glasses. Unless they have already experienced the early symptoms of presbyopia, patients tend to have a difficult time understanding the concept.

Laser Vision Correction Procedure: Summary of Patient Risks and Expectations

- Glasses may still be required.
- Presbyopia/reading glasses/monovision.
- Undercorrections.
- Overcorrections.
- Regression.
- Repeat surgery (enhancement).
- Infection.
- Night glare.

- Pain.
- Induced regular/irregular astigmatism.
- Loss of best corrected visual acuity.
- Qualitative vision loss: ghost images, monocular diplopia.

Candidate Selection

Patients, at the time of this writing, should be at least 18 years of age for correction of myopia. LASIK is capable of treating myopia as high as –30 D, which is many times in excess of what most potential candidates require for visual correction. The limit is really determined by the patient's corneal thickness or how much tissue is able to be removed and still leave the cornea thick enough to be healthy. The lower refractive limit for which LASIK is the preferred procedure is controversial, primarily because of the variability in surgeon comfort and skill levels with this relatively new procedure. If a surgeon achieves excellent results safely with PRK for mild and moderate myopia, the benefits of LASIK for these patients become more obscure. Some surgeons reserve LASIK for patients with more than –4.00 D, and some surgeons perform LASIK for all refractive procedures, even for corrections as low as 0.50–0.75 D of myopia. In the past, the general consensus was that the distinct advantage of LASIK over PRK occurs over –6.00 D, with significant benefits occurring above –9.00 D. As surgeon comfort levels improve, LASIK is replacing PRK as the preferred procedure for all myopic astigmatic corrections.

Other elements independent of refractive error that are important when looking at candidate selection include orbit configuration as well as ocular and general health considerations. Candidates with small or deep-set orbits should be avoided or counseled that the procedure may have to be aborted if the microkeratome ring cannot be well positioned or if proper suction is not obtainable. Other refractive procedures, such as PRK, can be considered as an alternative. Narrow palpebral fissures may also complicate placement of the suction ring and interfere with passage of the microkeratome. Any obstacles preventing smooth passage of the microkeratome will undoubtedly compromise the success of obtaining a good corneal flap and result in a higher complication rate. Patients with narrow palpebral openings or small orbits may experience increased discomfort intraoperatively and should be forewarned. There are new microkeratomes being developed, such as the Hansatome (Chiron), which is preferable for patients with flat corneas and small or deep-set orbits.

Other Considerations

Other ocular conditions that should be specifically examined preoperatively include corneal vascularization or pannus, which can result in intraoperative bleeding after the lamellar cut. Neovascularization may be a common finding among contact lens wearers. Many refractive surgery candidates are contact lens intolerant or are former extended-wear patients. Extended-wear patients who have dropped out of contact lenses may have neovascularization as a complication of wear. Although neovascularization is not an absolute contraindication, measures need to be taken to reduce intraoperative complications, and it would be wise to discuss this with the patient.[1,2]

Also, patients with flat corneas (mean keratometry, <41 D) produce small corneal flaps, and a free cap may be more common. To compensate and avoid this difficulty, the microkeratome will have to be adjusted to create a larger hinge.

Treating patients with a history of ocular surgery, including cataract, penetrating keratoplasty, and vitreoretinal surgery, should be avoided or approached with caution. Unless the surgeon has considerable experience, it can be difficult to achieve adequate suction pressure throughout the microkeratome cut, and an irregular thin flap may be obtained. For patients with PKP, the procedure should be placed on hold until 2 years after the surgery. Patients with a trabeculectomy and thin bleb should probably not have LASIK; instead, PRK should be considered.

For patients with recurrent erosion syndrome, superficial corneal scarring, or anterior basement membrane dystrophy, PRK may be the treatment of choice. The laser can be used to focally treat the superficial area of concern. Surface ablation offers these patients specific benefits in improving epithelial adhesion or eliminating superficial opacities. Also, poor epithelial adherence complicates lamellar surgery (LASIK) significantly, because it increases the incidence of epithelial ingrowth dramatically. Finally, treating patients with active ocular pathology, infection, or inflammation should be avoided.

LASIK is considered preferable to PRK for any patient who requires rapid visual rehabilitation, although the Laser-scrape technique of epithelial removal during PRK has reduced recovery time to as little as 24-hour re-epithelialization for some patients. True keloid formers are at a higher risk of developing haze after PRK, but there have been successful PRK procedures performed on patients who claim they are keloid formers. A *keloid former* is one who forms a mass of hyperplastic scar tissue after trauma; surgery; a burn; or severe cutaneous disease, such as cystic acne, and is more common in blacks. Generally, if these patients insist they want laser surgery, they should have LASIK. They should be counseled about the greater risks associated with their condition. Absolute contraindications for PRK and LASIK include active autoimmune diseases and collagen vascular diseases. These patients have an elevated risk of stromal melt with an exposed stromal surface.

With LASIK, because the epithelium remains intact and the stroma is only exposed intraoperatively, the concerns for precipitating a stromal melt are lessened. A number of patients with inactive lupus erythematosus have had LASIK performed and experienced an uncomplicated recovery without ocular sequelae. Treating patients with any active or severe vasculitic conditions should be avoided for any refractive surgery procedure, as these procedures are elective.

Another group of patients who are preferably treated with LASIK rather than PRK are those who are noncompliant or who exhibit medication intolerance. Steroid responders or those with a strong family history of glaucoma may be better suited for LASIK, because a steroid-induced pressure rise may seriously complicate the postoperative course or result in glaucomatous nerve cell death. Treatment of patients with diagnosed glaucomatous field loss should be avoided because raising the suction pressure even for a brief period with LASIK could further precipitate field loss. However, some experts believe this is controversial for cases of mild glaucoma, because the suction time is less than 1 minute. Patients with lifestyle issues, such as traveling in the near future for prolonged periods of time, may be better served with LASIK. Many patients simply want the convenience of LASIK.

Corneal Pachymetry

All patients need to have corneal pachymetry performed before the procedure to ensure that an adequate stromal bed thickness exists. Pachymetry of the entire cornea and knowledge of the epithelial thickness alone are important because the thickness of the cornea preoperatively affects the clinical response to procedures. For example, when evaluating a patient for an enhancement, if the corneal thickness reading is higher than expected, then the difference is due to a thickened epithelium. If the cornea is not thick enough for LASIK, PRK should be presented as an alternative, with appropriate risks being discussed. If a total corneal thickness less than or equal to 360 mm remains, or a stromal bed thickness of less than 250 mm remains, progressive corneal ectasia may be observed. The postoperative minimum total corneal thickness should be at least 360 mm, and ideally 400 mm, with at least a 250-mm stromal bed to ensure long-term stability. In other words, no greater than 50% of the corneal thickness should be penetrated to ensure long-term stability. For example, if a 160-micrometer flap is created on a 560-micrometer cornea, this would leave 400 microns in the stromal bed. The maximum ablation depth is 150 micrometers, which would leave the bed with 250 microns. Many lasers remove an average between 10.5–13.0 mm per D of correction, but this is dependent on the optical zone size and amount of correction. A generally safe rule of thumb is using 12 mm per diopter of correction[6] (see Chapter 8, LASIK Complications and Management, and Chapter 9, Outcomes).

Hyperopia

The upper limit of hyperopia presently imposed by the U.S. Food and Drug Administration (FDA) at this time of writing is +6.00 D. Because the curvature of the stromal bed increases secondary to the hyperopic ablation pattern, the ability to realign the corneal flap when treating higher degrees of correction is limited. Many surgeons choose not to treat over +4.00 D, as amounts higher than this are more likely to produce irregular astigmatism, and loss of best corrected acuity, and need multiple enhancements. Studies have shown low degrees of hyperopia being adequately treated with PRK, but LASIK appears to be the preferred treatment. The two main reasons are faster recovery time and stability of the hyperopic ablation pattern beneath the corneal flap. Another alternative in low hyperopia is laser thermokeratoplasty. At the time of this writing, LTK was approved by the FDA (see Chapter 11, Future Techniques and Investigational Procedures).

A procedure for hyperopia is considered successful when the patient is within 0.75 D of residual refractive error. Because many patients with lower degrees of hyperopia can see 20/40 uncorrected, it is best to speak to them about final refractive results versus acuity. This practice is especially true for younger patients. With patients with higher amounts of hyperopia, the treatment should be discussed in terms of the reduction in the degree of hyperopia. The ideal is less than 1 D of residual hyperopia remaining.

Patients typically will have a multifocal cornea postoperatively and will often see better at distance and near without correction. The multifocal effect comes from the multizone ablation. This effect is also seen with higher myopes but is not as easily detected by the patient. Higher myopes require more ablation zones than lower myopes, lending to a greater multifocal effect. Hyperopes appreciate the multifocal effect much more than myopes. Monovision is an option, so long as +6.00 D is not required in the near eye, which approaches the upper limit of LASIK.

Contraindications

Compared with PRK, LASIK has fewer contraindications involving wound healing. Systemic contraindications are almost nonexistent, with only a few ocular contraindications. One group of patients that is always contraindicated for elective refractive surgery is monocular patients. Keratoconus is a contraindication for refractive surgery at this time. Many surgeons will not operate on forme fruste keratoconus. However, many cases of forme fruste keratoconus have been performed with acceptable results. The concern is that true keratoconus will later develop, because ectasia has occurred in thinned corneas after LASIK. For forme fruste keratoconus, stromal thickness must be determined by corneal pachymetry. Young patients who may develop clinical keratoconus are specifically contraindicated. Once again, it is best to avoid treating any patients with active autoimmune disease; for patients with inactive autoimmune and collagen vascular disorders, however, LASIK is an acceptable procedure.

Undercorrected and overcorrected RK is not a contraindication to LASIK, however, there is a risk that the flap will separate at the incision sites. The greater the number of incisions, the greater the risk. These patients also cannot have a second LASIK procedure involving a recut of the flap, as it greatly increases the chance of flap fragmentation. PRK may be preferable in specific multiple incision cases. Surface ablation after RK, however, is associated with a five- to tenfold increase in haze formation and at least a 20% reduction in refractive predictability.

Observed reactions in RK patients range anywhere from achieving the desired correction targeted, to no change, to triple the correction input. After RK, the corneal instability produced makes it difficult to predict results. The two primary factors producing regression after PRK enhancement of RK are epithelial hyperplasia and haze formation. The advantage of LASIK over PRK for this subset of patients is the virtual elimination of both of these regression factors. LASIK gives a more predictable result than surface ablation because of the unaltered status of the epithelium. LASIK on a post-RK eye should be performed after a minimum 1-year RK incision healing period. Earlier penetrating keratoplasty is not contraindicated, but it should be performed at least 2 years after the surgery. This waiting period is to ensure wound stability and to prevent wound rupture or dehiscence when the microkeratome and suction ring are applied to the grafted eye. However, the standard nomograms may not be applicable to post-PKP patients, and irregular astigmatism cannot be corrected with current FDA-approved lasers. Earlier lamellar surgery, such as ALK (automated lamellar keratoplasty), is not a contraindication. A history of retinal tears or retinal detachment does not contraindicate LASIK.

LASIK Avoidance

Once again, patients to be avoided but not absolutely contraindicated for LASIK are ones with epithelial adherence problems or anterior basement membrane dystrophy. If the epithelial surface becomes denuded either partially or fully due to the microkeratome pass or perioperative medication, there is an increased risk of epithelial ingrowth and slower visual recovery. Conditions that alter the conjunctiva significantly, such as pterygium or conjunctival scars, could interfere with the ability to obtain and maintain adequate suction during the lamellar cut. This could increase the risk of a thin or perforated corneal flap.

Also, any condition that results in significant vitreous syneresis, including vitrectomy or pathological myopia (e.g., scleral buckle), may result in inadequate suction pressure intraoperatively. An experienced lamellar surgeon may attempt these more challenging cases, but the complication rate is higher. If the myopia level is appropriate for the procedure, PRK would be preferable.

Preoperative Examination

The following are tests important for preprocedure evaluation of the LASIK patient.

Visual Acuity

Just as visual acuity is important to document in all eye examinations, uncorrected and best corrected visual acuity must be documented. Extreme and severe myopia can be associated with reduced best corrected visual acuity. Best corrected acuity may differ between contact lens and spectacle correction. As mentioned before, patients who wear rigid gas-permeable contact lenses may experience a level of visual acuity that may be impossible to replicate with current forms of refractive surgery. Discussion and documentation of the discussion of these more-challenging cases is important. Patient satisfaction levels will be higher if patients have realistic expectations. Patients may not be suitable candidates if they have reduced acuity in one eye at a level below 20/40. If there were complications with the better eye, there is a risk that the patient's lifestyle could be adversely affected by restricted driving privileges.

Refraction

Very careful cycloplegic and manifest refractions must be performed with attention given to true vertex distance in cases of high myopia. Many times, higher myopes are overcorrected in their spectacle correction in an attempt to improve their quality of vision. Great care should be taken to obtain the correct refraction in these cases. In cases of extreme myopia, it might be prudent to fit the patient with a disposable contact lens for –8.00 to –10.00 D and then over-refract the patient. Always think of obtaining the least minus or the most plus power to decrease the possibility of over-correction.

Pearl:
For high myopia, fit a –8.00 to –10.00 disposable lens and over-refract to increase accuracy.

Anterior Segment Examination

Preoperative anterior segment examination is essential to rule out pre-existing pathology. Lids and lashes must be assessed for uncontrolled blepharitis, which should be treated preoperatively. Corneal clarity, vascularization from contact lens use, previous scars, evidence of keratoconus, endothelial changes, and hereditary dystrophies should all be evaluated and documented. If any lens changes are seen, it is important not only to document, but also to discuss the changes with the patient. Any significant changes to the lens should be evaluated, especially in high myopia, to assess whether it would be wise to wait and see if performing a lens extraction would be preferable to having laser vision correction. Any abnormalities seen, no matter how benign, should be documented and discussed with the patient to ensure the patient is aware of them preoperatively. Intraocular pressure should be documented preoperatively as a baseline to identify pre-existing pathology before topical steroid use. This is more important to consider with PRK.

Pearl:
If there are any lenticular changes present in high myopia, it may be better to delay LASIK and correct the refractive error later with an intraocular lens.

Another consideration in the preoperative examination is pupil size in dim light, because pupillary size and degree of myopia are the most important risk factors in night visual disturbances (i.e., glare, halos, starbursting). Patients with higher corrections and larger pupils should have at least a 6-mm optical zone treated. A 7-mm zone would be even better. Remember, the larger the optic zone, the more tissue is removed. Patients should be informed accordingly.

Corneal Topography

Preoperative corneal topography is important in planning laser vision correction and has clearly become the accepted standard of care. It helps to plan surgery and also to identify the changes that have been created postoperatively. It is effective in identifying early keratoconus and *forme fruste* varieties of keratoconus. There are various clinical features for identifying keratoconus, keratoconus suspects, and variants. In fact, corneal topography is probably the gold standard for diagnosing keratoconus. The two primary features observed with keratoconus are corneal steepening and asymmetry. In keratoconus, inferior and occasionally central corneal steepening of 47 D or greater, asymmetry between the inferior and superior aspects of the same cornea, and asymmetry between the two eyes are commonly observed. One must be able to understand how topography works to read a map effectively. It is based on reflections from the corneal surface that have been digitized and transformed to color codes that indicate changes in curvature. Current placido-based technology is good, but more advanced systems, such as slit lamp rasterography, are quickly entering the market.

Topography also allows us to understand a number of postoperative surgical parameters and problems, such as irregular astigmatism, central islands, and decentered ablations. Systems such as the Orbscan (Bausch & Lomb, Rochester, NY) and future topographers are able to give us more information, such as posterior corneal curvature, central corneal thickness, and peripheral corneal thickness. If the patient is a contact lens wearer, topography is invaluable (see Chapter 5, Preoperative Management of Contact Lens Wearing LASIK Candidates).

Retinal Examination

It is imperative that a dilated retinal examination be performed, and the patient must understand that the risk of retinal detachment does not decrease simply because his or her dependence on glasses or contact lenses decreases. High myopes are generally at greater risk for posterior segment pathology. As stated before, patients must continue with annual eye examinations, and this need must be stressed to them. Patients tend to get the idea that because their vision is corrected, they are no longer at risk for complications associated with myopia. Peripheral retinal pathology, macular staphylomas, posterior staphylomas, and myopic degeneration should be documented and discussed with the patient.

Candidate Preparation

To properly prepare the candidate for laser vision correction, other specific issues to address once he or she has completed the consultative process and preoperative examination include contact lens wear and the timing of the second eye.

Contact Lens Wear

The patient must discontinue contact lens wear with sufficient time preoperatively to allow the natural contour of the cornea to be re-established. With LASIK, it is not quite as important for the cornea to recover before the procedure as it is with PRK. For patients who have a long history of contact lens use, it is important to allow a longer period for recovery (see Chapter 5, Preoperative Management of Contact Lens Wearing LASIK Candidates).

Timing of the Second Eye

Many patients seek bilateral simultaneous surgery, and the risks and benefits should be conservatively evaluated for each patient. The benefits are convenience and little disruption of work and lifestyle. Additionally, if surgery on both eyes is performed simultaneously, anxiety is reduced and side effects related to night glare and anisometropia are minimized. Surgeons report that patients experience less night vision problems with a bilateral, as opposed to unilateral, procedure.

Risks of bilateral surgery are based on the degree of myopia, the refractive predictability, and the complication rate for that group. Most patients do not believe that they will incur a complication; they readily accept the risk of bilateral infections, haze, or other healing problems. Refractive complications present problems, especially with overcorrections. Special consideration must be given to blurred vision bilaterally, with an inability to drive and perhaps work for 1 to 2 weeks while the refraction stabilizes.

Bilateral Simultaneous Surgery

Disadvantages of bilateral simultaneous surgery are the following:

- Bilateral complications: infections, haze
- Inability to compensate nomogram for improper refractive outcome with second eye
- Bilateral undercorrections
- Bilateral overcorrections
- Bilateral loss of best corrected vision

Advantages of bilateral simultaneous surgery are the following:

- Improved patient convenience
- Possible reduced anxiety (no need to return for second eye)
- Improved subjective vision (unable to compare to contact lens)
- Balance restored rapidly
- Night glare improved rapidly

References

1. Machat JJ. Excimer Laser Refractive Surgery: Practice and Principles. Thorofare, NJ: Slack, 1996.
2. Machat JJ, Slade SG, Probst LE (eds). The Art of LASIK (2nd ed). Thorofare, NJ: Slack, 1999.
3. Gimbel HV, Penno EEA. Early Postoperative Complications: 24 to 48 Hours. In HV Gimbel, EEA Penno (eds), LASIK Complications. Thorofare, NJ: Slack, 1999.
4. Hom MM. Monovision and LASIK. J Am Optom Assoc 1999;70:117–122.
5. Lingua RW. The Essentials of LASIK and Its Co-Management. Brea, California: TLC Laser Center, 1997.
6. Nagy ZZ, Hiscott P, Seitz B, et al. Ultraviolet-B enhances corneal stromal response to 193-nm excimer laser treatment. Ophthalmology 1997;104:375–380.

CHAPTER 5

Preoperative Management of Contact Lens–Wearing LASIK Candidates

Arthur B. Epstein

Although contact lens wearers are among the most likely candidates for refractive surgery, they also present a variety of clinical challenges and potential pitfalls.[1,2] This chapter examines the possible complications of refractive surgery in the context of contact lens wear and explores strategies to prevent unexpected outcomes. Special attention is directed to identifying patients at risk for possible problems.

Corneal and Refractive Stability

Surgical procedures, such as LASIK, that permanently alter the corneal surface require refractive and topographic stability to assure a predictable postoperative endpoint. Caution must be exercised with the contact lens-wearing patient because lens wear can induce transient, as well as permanent, topographic and refractive changes that patients are often unaware of.[3–7] Furthermore, these changes can be occult and unpredictable and their resolution typically indeterminate.[7] In some cases, contact lens–induced corneal distortion can be extremely severe.[6] Only when complete histories before contact lens wear are available can stability be confirmed with relative certainty.

The risks of performing surgery on an unstable patient with an unknown baseline refractive error or topographic profile can be considerable. If undiscovered, contact lens–induced changes may inadvertently and permanently result in postsurgical corneal surface irregularity. This may manifest as irregular astigmatism, significant under- or overcorrection, or refractive instability. To prevent such mishaps, the preoperative evaluation of the contact lens wearer should be directed toward ensuring predictability and stability. Specific areas of concern include the following:

45

- Contact lens–induced corneal distortion and irregular astigmatism
- Occult keratoconus or other corneal ectatic condition
- Occult shift in refractive state
- Relative refractive instability (indeterminate endpoint)
- Physical conditions unrelated to contact lens wear that may cause temporary refractive shifts, such as floppy eyelid syndrome, lid imbrication syndrome, or chalazion

In addition, rigid lens wearers, patients wearing thick, low Dk hydrophilic lenses, those on extended-wear schedules and patients with a history of lens-related corneal warpage should be approached with greater caution.

Corneal Warpage and Irregular Astigmatism

Although corneal warpage has classically been associated with polymethylmethacrylate (PMMA) lenses, distortion of the corneal surface may occur with all types of contact lenses.[3,6,7] Potential causes of refractive and corneal curvature changes in contact lens wearers include mechanical forces applied by the contact lens and prolonged hypoxia.[8] The greatest shifts have been reported in PMMA wearers.[7] Clinical findings such as central corneal clouding (Figure 5.1), edematous corneal formations and endothelial changes are ubiquitous in PMMA lens wearers. Temporary or permanent refractive shifts evident on lens removal, termed *spectacle blur*, are characterized by corneal distortion and irregular astigmatism that can no longer

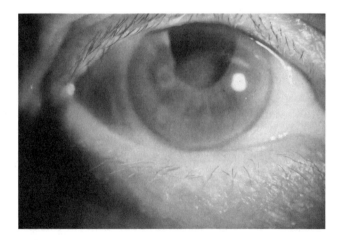

FIGURE 5.1. Central corneal clouding associated with polymethylmethacrylate lens wear.

be corrected with spectacles. During the heyday of PMMA lens wear, spectacle blur was a frequent and disconcerting problem that plagued both PMMA lens wearers and doctors, who often had to remake spectacles.

A variety of strategies were devised to manage PMMA hard lens–wearing patients with transient spectacle blur who desired occasional spectacle wear.[9,10] In this author's experience, the most successful approach entailed determining when and for how long patients wished to wear spectacles. Patients were then instructed to return for refraction at the approximate time of day they wished to wear spectacles. They were also told to remove their contact lenses sufficiently before the examination to allow the refraction to occur at the approximate midpoint of the desired spectacle-wearing time. Although this technique produced acceptable spectacle prescriptions, its precision is inadequate for a presurgical evaluation.

The effects of contact lenses on the cornea have fascinated researchers for decades. Beginning in the 1960s, Rengstorff extensively investigated refractive and topographic changes associated with contact lenses.[11,12] Although now primarily of historical significance, the classic *Rengstorff graph* plotted refractive change after discontinuation of PMMA lens wear over time.[13] Rengstorff demonstrated that a relatively stable return to baseline occurred at approximately 21 days after cessation of rigid gas-permeable (RGP) lens wear. His later work explored corneal changes associated with RGP and soft contact lenses.[14,15]

Modern rigid lenses span a large range of physiologic performance characteristics and produce significant variation in clinical effects on the cornea. Additionally, interpersonal differences in oxygen requirements and response to general and regional hypoxia play a significant, but individualized role in corneal changes precipitated by contact lens wear. In general, properly fitted RGP lenses tend to cause minimal refractive and topographic change.[16] However, lower Dk materials and lenses that are habitually decentered can predispose to corneal warpage.[8]

Although PMMA and RGP lenses are most frequently associated with corneal distortion, soft lenses can also induce significant refractive and topographic change (see Color Plate 1).[7,17,18] Topographic changes in soft lens wearers can mimic keratoconus (Figure 5.2) or assume unusual patterns (Figure 5.3). Soft lens–induced corneal alterations may also be subtle and appear independent of edema and overall corneal thickness change.[19] Regional differences in oxygen transmissibility and subsequent physiologic effects on the cornea can be significant, especially in high minus or high plus-powered soft lenses (Figure 5.4).[20,21] This may be a causative factor in soft lens–induced corneal distortion. Dry eye may contribute to this effect by further altering lens transmissibility.[22] Because soft lenses are not generally believed to induce these changes, they can present a hidden, yet significant, source of risk for unexpected outcomes in refractive surgery candidates.

Special lenses can cause unique problems. Annular tinted lenses have been reported to induce a peculiar ring-shaped pattern of transient corneal

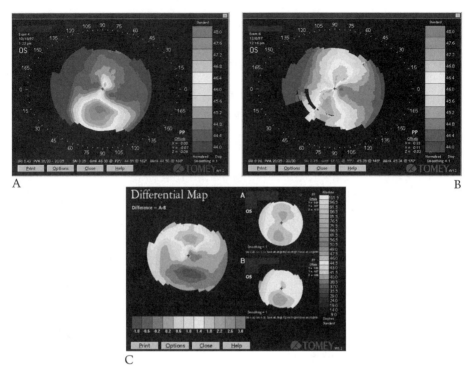

FIGURE 5.2. **(A, B)** Serial topographies of soft lens–induced corneal warpage mimicking keratoconus. Note the resolution over a 2-month period. **(C)** Difference map above using absolute scale, showing 7 diopters of topographic change.

warpage and irregular astigmatism.[23,24] This appears to be related to the thickness of the lens pigment and resolves rapidly once lens wear is discontinued. Prism-ballasted soft toric lenses can cause regional corneal warpage, typically reflected by inferior steepening or an increase in with-the-rule corneal astigmatism (Figure 5.5).

Keratoconus Detection

Most authorities consider keratoconus a contraindication to refractive surgery, including LASIK. Paradoxically, due to self selection, the patient population seeking refractive surgery may contain a disproportionately large number of patients with keratoconus and other topographic anomalies.[25,26] Keratoconus corneas are believed to have altered biochemical or mechanical properties that may lead to unpredictable refractive outcomes in patients with the disorder.[27,28] Although some reports suggest otherwise,

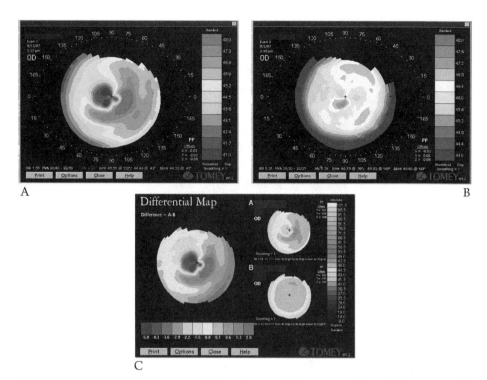

FIGURE 5.3. (**A, B**) Serial topographies of corneal distortion induced by a 4-year-old daily-wear soft lens. Note the resolution over approximately 1 month. (**C**) Difference map of above using absolute scale showing resolution.

prudence dictates that keratoconus patients be identified and advised against having LASIK and other refractive procedures.[29–31]

The advent of videokeratography has made it possible to detect subclinical keratoconus with comparative ease. Routine preoperative topographic screening for refractive surgery has uncovered a significant number of refractive surgery candidates with subclinical or forme fruste keratoconus, irregular astigmatism or contact lens–related corneal distortion.[25,32]

Because keratoconus is a permanent condition and contact lens–induced corneal warpage is typically transient, it is important to differentiate between the two.[7] Most patients with contact lens–related distortion need only be patient while their condition resolves. They may then undergo refractive surgery. Keratoconus patients should be counseled about their disorder and its possible progression. The current standard of care dictates that they be advised of the risks of undergoing refractive surgery procedures.

Contact lens–induced warpage and true keratoconus exhibit similar corneal topographic patterns. However, they demonstrate two uniquely dif-

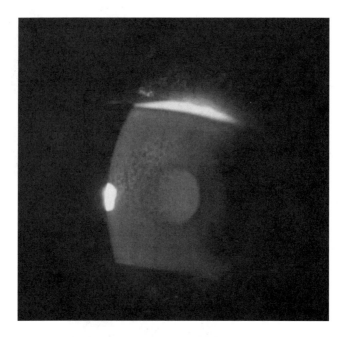

FIGURE 5.4. Corneal epithelial edema in a soft lens wearer caused by a low-Dk plus-powered lens—a probable factor in corneal warpage.

ferent geometric shapes that can be readily and accurately differentiated using the various corneal shaped indices of videokeratoscopy.[33] In addition, most contact lens–related corneal warpage shows signs of resolution within weeks of discontinuing lens wear, whereas true keratoconus tends to be more stable and can be progressive.

Keratoconus, subclinical keratoconus (forme fruste), contact lens–induced inferior corneal steepening, a displaced corneal apex and pellucid marginal degeneration all produce relatively similar corneal topography maps that demonstrate superior corneal flattening and marked inferior corneal steepening. Some topography systems (e.g., Humphrey Systems [Dublin, CA], Tomey Technology [Cambridge, MA], and Dicon [San Diego, CA]) have introduced keratoconus detection software that attempts to detect and possibly differentiate these conditions. For example, Humphrey Systems' PathFinder Software Module for the Atlas Corneal Topographer differentiates *normal, corneal distortion, subclinical keratoconus* and *keratoconus* by statistically analyzing three indices (the shape factor, corneal irregularity measure, and toric mean reference curvature) and comparing them to a normative database. Tomey Technology uses an artificial intelligence expert system to determine the presence, absence, and degree of keratoconus based on the analysis of a series of topographically derived numeric indices. Dicon

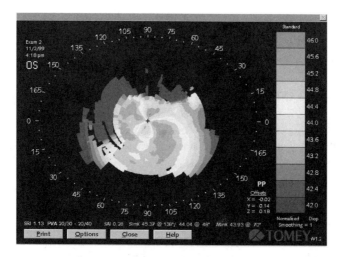

FIGURE 5.5. Corneal topography of corneal warpage from a poorly fitted, prism-ballasted, soft toric contact lens.

uses an analysis of apex localization using tangential maps to predict the probability of keratoconus.

Contact Lens–Induced Occult Refractive Shifts

Because contact lens wear can differentially, but evenly, change the shape of the underlying cornea, it can affect a patient's refractive status without inducing obvious topographic irregularity or causing irregular astigmatism. In fact, this is the basis of *orthokeratology*, which produces a generally predictable, but mostly transient, change in corneal shape and refraction.[34–37]

In rigid lens wearers, refractive change appears, due in part to a redistribution of corneal tissue.[38] Long-term contact lens–induced hypoxia has been implicated in the modification of epithelial cell production and epithelial thinning, and in the rate of cell desquamation.[39,40] Mechanical factors are likely to play a role as well.

Changes in corneal thickness and refraction have also been noted in soft contact lens wearers.[41–43] Edema may play a role; however, edema-induced thickness changes do not necessarily correlate with observed refractive changes.[16] Increases in myopia are frequently observed in patients soon after initiating low-Dk soft contact lens wear. This has been termed *myopic creep* and may be, at least in part, transient. Even with soft contact lenses, in which mechanical factors would be relatively minor, the lens-cornea fitting relationship may play a role in precipitating refractive change.[44] Lid forces acting on the differential thickness of the contact lenses can be an effective force for reshaping the cornea (Figure 5.6). In presbyopic contact lens wearers, another factor that must be considered is the effect of monovision, which can cause an anisometropic refractive shift.[45]

Refractive Instability

Although contact lenses can effect significant changes in corneal refraction and shape, under normal circumstances they do not cause significant refractive or topographic instability. However, when a contact lens remodels the corneal surface, a period of relative instability ensues as the induced change resolves. Because the magnitude of the change and the time course for complete resolution cannot readily be determined, stability remains uncertain until confirmed by serial topography and refraction.[5,7] Resolution can take several weeks to many months.[7] Obvious cases of lens-related corneal warpage should not be difficult to detect; however, subtle cases may be less apparent, leading to an inappropriate refractive endpoint determination.

Other non–contact lens–related causes of refractive instability could affect contact lens wearers. These include unstable diabetes, nuclear cata-

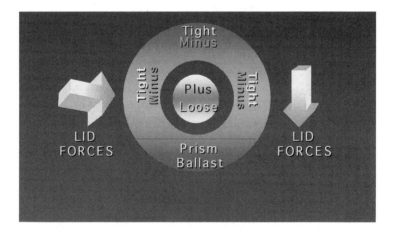

FIGURE 5.6. Diagram showing the corneal effects of contact lens bearing forces. This diagram demonstrates the forces applied by lid movement (both down and in) through the lens to the cornea. Minus-powered lenses are thicker in the periphery and thus apply more force to the peripheral cornea. Plus-powered lenses are thicker in the center and more bearing occurs in that area. Prism-ballasted lenses tend to effect the peripheral cornea because of the increased thickness in that area. In addition, loosely-fitted lenses tend to bear centrally, whereas tight lenses primarily bear in the periphery.

ract, accommodative spasm or paralysis, Marfan's syndrome, myasthenia gravis, and drug or medication effects. It is important to consider these possibilities in exploring possible causes of unanticipated refractive change in a contact lens wearer.

Physical Conditions Unrelated to Contact Lens Wear That May Cause Temporary Refractive Change

A variety of lid abnormalities and disorders, such as chalazia, can induce refractive changes.[46–48] These changes affect both the contact lens wearer and the non–contact lens wearer, and typically persist until the cause is removed. Astigmatism is most common, although spherical changes, such as induced hyperopia, have been reported.[49] With astigmatic changes, minus cylinder axes are consistently oriented 90 degrees away from the lesion, and generally resolve with resolution of the lesion.[47] Vernal keratoconjunctivitis and severe giant papillary conjunctivitis have also been reported to induce refractive change.[50] In some cases, refractive changes caused by lid abnormalities appear permanent despite resolution of the lesion.[51]

Soft tissue defects of the lid can also create astigmatic errors. The presence of perilimbal masses, as well as their removal, can induce astigmatism.[52] Forces at or near the corneoscleral limbus can produce changes in corneal curvature, resulting in increased astigmatism. There is a shift of the axis of astigmatism toward the meridian, 90 degrees away from the external force, or an increase of astigmatism along the meridian at which the force was exerted.[53]

Ptyergia, although generally obvious on ophthalmic examination, can induce astigmatic changes before invasion of the visual axis while patients are still wearing contact lenses. Ptyergia typically induce with-the-rule astigmatism, which can be visually significant early in their course despite appearing innocuous.[54] It is important to ensure that the lids and ocular adnexa are thoroughly examined during the preoperative examination.

Preoperative Examination of the Contact Lens Wearer

A variety of strategies for preoperatively managing the contact lens wearer have been recommended. The specific approach is generally dependent on the type of contact lens worn and the length of lens wear experience.

Stable refraction and corneal topography are critical preoperative requirements. However, determining baseline stability is not always a simple or straightforward task. Several experts and laser surgery providers have attempted to simplify the process by recommending preset periods of lens discontinuation before the preoperative examination. These periods range from as little as 48 hours for soft lens wearers to several months for rigid lens wearers. Some suggest that the period of abstinence from lens wear be keyed to the relative length of previous wear; for example, some advise 4 weeks' abstinence for every decade of rigid lens wear.

Applying a fixed and inflexible approach to any aspect of clinical care is fraught with potential problems. Contact lenses can affect the cornea in a variety of ways. The time needed to achieve baseline stability and a consistent endpoint may be difficult to predict. Most contact lens wearers with topography and refraction readings within 0.50 diopters (D) of earlier values appear to stabilize quickly on lens discontinuation.[55] Rigid lens wearers reportedly stabilize within 5 weeks and soft lens wearers within 2 weeks of lens discontinuation. However, apparent stability is of little consolation to an individual patient with a poor surgical outcome that was caused by preoperative misjudgment.

Pearl:
Simply recommending preset periods of contact lens discontinuation is fraught with potential problems.

Computerized corneal topography can be a useful tool for evaluating the effects of contact lens wear. A significant number of prospective refractive surgery patients, especially contact lens wearers, have abnormal topography.[5,7] In one study of 106 eyes, 33% were found to have abnormal corneal topography.[25] Thirty-eight percent of contact lens wearers showed irregular astigmatism, loss of radial symmetry, or absence of the normal progressive flattening from the center to the periphery of the cornea. Rigid contact lens wearers are affected more often and more severely, especially when their lenses are habitually decentered.[8] As discussed earlier, a disproportionately high percentage of refractive surgery candidates have keratoconus, probably because of preselection.

Other than keratoconic-like patterns, examples of topographic shifts that should be screened for include shift from a prolate to an oblate shape, smile impression arcs, and variable irregular astigmatism. Serial topography and topographic difference maps generated by a consistent instrument on a given patient over time may reveal such subtle changes.

The normal cornea is a prolate shape, steeper in the center and flatter in the periphery. Long-term, flat-fitting lenses can permanently shift the cornea to an oblate pattern by flattening the central cornea and, secondarily, steepening the periphery. This type of warpage may not be detected with keratometry or manifest refraction if the astigmatism is regular and the patient remains correctable to 20/20.

RGP-induced, smile-like arcuate corneal shape changes are most often located in the inferior third of the cornea and can implicate a suboptimal fitting relationship. In traditional RGP fitting, a flattened arcuate compression ring usually signifies unintended corneal molding from the inferior edge of a superiorly decentered RGP. Just outside the lens edge, an arcuate zone of steepening appears, best viewed on an instantaneous map.

Other than detecting these abnormalities, the best use for computerized corneal topography is to evaluate the stability of the corneal surface. Stability can be assured by comparing serial topographies taken over a sufficiently long period until no further changes are evident. Topographic findings alone should not be relied on to confirm refractive stability. Topography should be interpreted only in the context of a complete clinical examination. Retinoscopy may also be used to subjectively evaluate the quality and homogeneity of the patient's optic system, including the corneal surface.

Another reliable indicator of stability is two or more serial refractions, performed a week apart, that are repeatable to within 0.25 D of the previous measurement. If results are uncertain or the patient is suspected of having possible occult problems, additional testing should be performed several days later to verify previous results. Ideally, the combination of repeatable refraction and serially stable topography offers the greatest assurance that any transient effects have resolved.

As a general rule, a final preoperative check performed the day before or the day of surgery is a good way to confirm stability in a previous contact lens wearer, regardless of mode of previous lens wear or problems.

Handling Special Situations

Previous rigid lens wear can present special problems in refractive surgery candidates. Some surgeons believe that the clarity that rigid lenses provide cannot be matched by currently available refractive surgery and that these patients are destined to be dissatisfied with refractive surgery results no matter how good the outcome.

Rigid lenses also have a much greater effect on the corneal surface, and these effects take longer to resolve.[7] Decentered rigid lenses, as discussed in the section Preoperative Examination of the Contact Lens Wearer, can produce severe and asymmetric corneal warpage that can take many months to resolve and, in some cases, may result in permanently decreased vision.[5,8,25]

Ideally, all patients should be weaned off rigid lenses slowly. This is especially important for those still wearing PMMA lenses, in which the sudden cessation of lens wear and the resultant mechanical and metabolic shifts may further undermine corneal instability. A large percentage of long-time PMMA wearers have some degree of corneal warpage.

The preoperative management of rigid lens patients who show signs of corneal warpage or instability can be problematic. The majority have significant prescription needs and will not be functional in the absence of adequate correction. Spectacles are impractical; the necessary frequent lens changes make the cost prohibitive. Refitting them with higher permeability rigid lenses may facilitate a more rapid return to stability. However, the value of this intermediate step remains unproved, especially with PMMA wearers.[56]

Disposable and frequent replacement soft lenses, although often providing only adequate vision, may serve as a temporary visual bridge during recovery.

In cases of severe warpage, frequent lens changes may be necessary. Many of these patients have significant astigmatism, which is why they were initially fitted with rigid lenses. These patients usually require toric soft lens correction. If rigid lenses were habitually high riding, inferior steepening may destabilize prism-ballasted toric lenses. In such cases, fitting a steeper base curve or a larger diameter may help to stabilize the lens. It may take many months for patients with corneal warpage to stabilize and for preoperative spectacle lens wear to become possible.

When no corneal warpage is evident, rigid lens wearers should discontinue lens wear and be followed until stability is confirmed by serial examination. Most rigid lens wearers stabilize within 3–6 weeks. Lower Dk lenses may require longer periods to achieve stability.

Extended-wear patients and patients who are otherwise subjected to chronic hypoxia experience a variety of corneal changes.[57] Extended wear also reduces stromal keratocyte density, which may affect healing after LASIK.[58] Prudence suggests that patients on extended-wear schedules be followed cautiously and that additional time be provided to ensure a return to baseline. Extended-wear patients should discontinue lens wear at least 3 weeks before their first preoperative examination. Reevaluation before surgery is especially important with extended-wear patients, because refractive and corneal shape changes may be subtle and difficult to detect.

Conclusion

In practice, refractive surgeons tend to trivialize the effect of contact lens wear. An Internet-based survey conducted on Keranet, a cornea specialist–specific mailing list, revealed that responding surgeons had patients discontinue soft lens wear for an average of 8.3 days and rigid lens wear for an average of 17.5 days before surgery. Only one responding surgeon reported performing serial refraction and topography to ensure stability before operating. At a time of increasing awareness of complications and less-than-ideal outcomes, it is interesting to speculate on how trivializing the role of contact lenses may be part of the genesis of some of these problems.

Pearl:
During a recent informal Internet study, only one surgeon reported performing serial refraction and topography to ensure corneal stability.

LASIK co-management offers an opportunity to focus on patient needs independent of the surgeon's involvement. This provides an additional opinion for the patient and, if performed diligently, can decrease risk. After all, two heads are better than one.

References

1. Migneco MK, Pepose JS. Attitudes of successful contact lens wearers toward refractive surgery. J Refract Surg 1996;12:128–133.
2. Naroo SA, Shah S, Kapoor R. Factors that influence patient choice of contact lens or photorefractive keratectomy. J Refract Surg 1999;15:132–136.
3. Hartstein J. Corneal warping due to wearing of corneal contact lenses. A report of 12 cases. Am J Ophthalmol 1965;60:1103–1104.
4. Hill JF. Variation in refractive error and corneal curvature after wearing hydrophilic contact lenses. J Am Optom Assoc 1975;46:1136–1138.
5. Ruiz-Montenegro J, Mafra CH, Wilson SE, et al. Corneal topographic alterations in normal contact lens wearers. Ophthalmology 1993;100:128–134.
6. Phillips CI. Contact lenses and corneal deformation: cause, correlate or coincidence? Acta Ophthalmol Scand Suppl 1990;68:661–668.
7. Wilson SE, Lin DT, Klyce SD, et al. Topographic changes in contact lens-induced corneal warpage. Ophthalmology 1990;97:734–744.
8. Wilson SE, Lin DT, Klyce SD, et al. Rigid contact lens decentration: a risk factor for corneal warpage. CLAO J 1990;16:177–182.
9. Bennett ES, Tomlinson A. A comparison of two techniques of refitting long-term polymethyl methacrylate contact lens wearers. Am J Optom Physiol Opt 1983;60:139–145.
10. Bennett ES. Immediate refitting with gas permeable lenses. J Am Optom Assoc 1983;54:239–242.
11. Rengstorff RH. Corneal curvature and astigmatic changes subsequent to contact lens wear. J Am Optom Assoc 1965;36:996–1000.
12. Rengstorff RH. The Fort Dix report: longitudinal study of the effects of contact lenses. Am J Optom 1965;42:153–163.
13. Hom MM. Thoughts on contact lens refractive changes. Contact Lens Forum 1986;11:16–20.
14. Rengstorff RH, Nilsson KT. Long-term effects of extended wear lenses: changes in refraction, corneal curvature, and visual acuity. Am J Optom Physiol Opt 1985;62:66–68.
15. Barnett WA, Rengstorff RH. Adaptation to hydrogel contact lenses: variations in myopia and corneal curvature measurements. J Am Optom Assoc 1977;48:363–366.
16. Sanaty M, Temel A. Corneal curvature changes in soft and rigid gas permeable contact lens wearers after two years of lens wear. CLAO J 1996;22:186–188.
17. Grosvenor T. Changes in corneal curvature and subjective refraction of soft contact lens wearers. Am J Optom Physiol Opt 1975;52:405–413.
18. Carney LG. Hydrophilic lens effects on central and peripheral corneal thickness and corneal topography. Am J Optom Physiol Opt 1975;52:521–523.
19. Rom ME, Keller WB, Meyer CJ, et al. Relationship between corneal edema and topography. CLAO J 1995;21:191–194.
20. Fatt I, Weissman BA, Ruben CM. Areal differences in oxygen supply to a cornea wearing an optically powered hydrogel contact lens. CLAO J 1993;19:226–234.

21. Fatt I. New physiological paradigms to assess the effect of lens oxygen transmissibility on corneal health. CLAO J 1996;22:25–29.

22. Efron N, Morgan PB. Hydrogel contact lens dehydration and oxygen transmissibility. CLAO J 1999;25:148–151.

23. Schanzer MC, Mehta RS, Arnold TP, et al. Irregular astigmatism induced by annular tinted contact lenses. CLAO J 1989;15:207–211.

24. Bucci FA Jr, Evans RE, Moody KJ, et al. The annular tinted contact lens syndrome: corneal topographic analysis of ring-shaped irregular astigmatism caused by annular tinted contact lenses. CLAO J 1997;23:161–167.

25. Wilson SE, Klyce SD. Screening for corneal topographic abnormalities before refractive surgery. Ophthalmology 1994;101:147–152.

26. Nesburn AB, Bahri S, Salz J, et al. Keratoconus detected by videokeratography in candidates for photorefractive keratectomy. J Refract Surg 1995;11: 194–201.

27. Saragoussi JJ, Pouliquen YJ. Does the progressive increasing effect of radial keratotomy (hyperopic shift) correlate with undetected early keratoconus? J Refract Surg 1994;10:45–48.

28. Seiler T, Quurke AW. Iatrogenic keratectasia after LASIK in a case of forme fruste keratoconus. J Cataract Refract Surg 1998;24:1007–1009.

29. Appiotti A, Gualdi M. Treatment of keratoconus with laser in situ keratomileusis, photorefractive keratectomy, and radial keratotomy. J Refract Surg 1999;15:S240–S242.

30. Kremer I, Shochot Y, Kaplan A, Blumenthal M. Three year results of photoastigmatic refractive keratectomy for mild and atypical keratoconus. J Cataract Refract Surg 1998;24:1581–1588.

31. Bowman CB, Thompson KP, Stulting RD. Refractive keratotomy in keratoconus suspects. J Refract Surg 1995;11:202–206.

32. Maeda N, Klyce SD, Tano Y. Detection and classification of mild irregular astigmatism in patients with good visual acuity. Surv Ophthalmol 1998;43:53–58.

33. Lebow KA, Grohe RM. Differentiating contact lens-induced warpage from true keratoconus using corneal topography. CLAO J 1999;25:114–122.

34. Kerns RL. Research in orthokeratology. Part IV: results and observations. J Am Optom Assoc 1977;48:227–238.

35. Polse KA, Brand RJ, Vastine DW, Schwalbe JS. Corneal change accompanying orthokeratology. Plastic or elastic? Results of a randomized controlled clinical trial. Arch Ophthalmol 1983;101:1873–1878.

36. Polse KA, Brand RJ, Schwalbe JS, et al. The Berkeley Orthokeratology Study, Part II: Efficacy and duration. Am J Optom Physiol Opt 1983;60:187–198.

37. Dave T, Ruston D. Current trends in modern orthokeratology. Ophthalmic Physiol Opt 1998;18:224–233.

38. Swarbrick HA, Wong G, O'Leary DJ. Corneal response to orthokeratology. Optom Vis Sci 1998;75:791–799.

39. Ren DH, Petroll WM, Jester JV, Cavanagh HD. The effect of rigid gas permeable contact lens wear on proliferation of rabbit corneal and conjunctival epithelial cells. CLAO J 1999;25:136–141.

40. Ren DH, Petroll WM, Jester JV, et al. The relationship between contact lens oxygen permeability and binding of *Pseudomonas aeruginosa* to human corneal epithelial cells after overnight and extended wear. CLAO J 1999;25: 80–100.
41. Hovding G. Variations of refractive error during the first year of contact lens wear. Acta Ophthalmol Scand Suppl 1983;61:129–140.
42. Grosvenor T. Changes in corneal curvature and subjective refraction of soft contact lens wearers. Am J Optom Physiol Opt 1975;52:405–413.
43. Hill JF. Variation in refractive error and corneal curvature after wearing hydrophilic contact lenses. J Am Optom Assoc 1975;46:1136–1138.
44. Hill JF. Changes in corneal curvature and refractive error upon refitting with flatter hydrophilic contact lenses. J Am Optom Assoc 1976;47:1214–1216.
45. Wick B, Westin E. Change in refractive anisometropia in presbyopic adults wearing monovision contact lens correction. Optom Vis Sci 1999;76:33–39.
46. Langmann A, Lindner S. Normalization of asymmetric astigmatism after intralesional steroid injection for upper eye lid hemangioma in childhood. Doc Ophthalmol 1994;87:283–290.
47. Bogan S, Simon JW, Krohel GB, Nelson LB. Astigmatism associated with adnexal masses in infancy. Arch Ophthalmol 1987;105:1368–1370.
48. Diamond S. Pathology of the refracting media which influences the refraction of the eye. Opt J Rev Optom 1950;87:35.
49. Santa Cruz CS, Culotta T, Cohen EJ, Rapuano CJ. Chalazion-induced hyperopia as a cause of decreased vision. Ophthalmic Surg Lasers 1997;28:683–684.
50. Tabbara KF. Ocular complications of vernal keratoconjunctivitis. Can J Ophthalmol 1999;34:88–92.
51. Robb RM. Refractive errors associated with hemangiomas of the eyelids and orbit in infancy. Am J Ophthalmol 1977;83:52–58.
52. Budak K, Khater TT, Friedman NJ, Koch DD. Corneal topographic changes induced by excision of perilimbal lesions. Ophthalmic Surg Lasers 1999;30: 458–464.
53. Cuttone JM, Durso F, Miller M, Evans LS. The relationship between soft tissue anomalies around the orbit and globe and astigmatic refractive errors: a preliminary report. J Pediatr Ophthalmol Strabismus 1980;17:29–36.
54. Lin A, Stern G. Correlation between pterygium size and induced corneal astigmatism. Cornea 1998;17:28–30.
55. Budak K, Hamed AM, Friedman NJ, Koch DD. Preoperative screening of contact lens wearers before refractive surgery. J Cataract Refract Surg 1999;25: 1080–1086.
56. Novo AG, Pavlopoulos G, Feldman ST. Corneal topographic changes after refitting polymethylmethacrylate contact lens wearers into rigid gas permeable materials. CLAO J 1995;21:47–51.
57. Epstein AB. The current state of extended wear. Contact Lens Spectrum 1999;14:19–22.
58. Jalbert I, Stapleton F. Effect of lens wear on corneal stroma: preliminary findings. Aust N Z J Ophthalmol 1999;27:211–213.

CHAPTER 6

Description of Primary Procedure and Retreatment

Milton M. Hom and Robert W. Lingua

Apply suction, check pressure, wet, then cut.
—Jeffrey J. Machat

The LASIK surgical procedure can vary from surgeon to surgeon. Every surgeon chooses and refines their own technique.[1] Because of the rapid advancements in technology, the procedure itself continues to improve. Although the procedure will probably change by the time you read this, the concepts should generally be the same.

Laser Room

The laser room environment should be set up for optimal performance. The room is kept between 18° and 24° C. Humidity should be stable and below 50%. Any variations in humidity and temperature can change the outcomes (see Chapter 9, Outcomes). Several air filtration units should be in use to keep the atmosphere surgically clean.[2,3] A well-placed fan can help to dissipate the odor of ablated cornea, which patients often find disturbing.[4] The procedure takes approximately 5 minutes in the hands of an experienced surgeon.[5]

Medications

Before the procedure, patients normally receive a mild sedative, such as alprazolam (Xanax), to reduce anxiety. The sedative also allows the patient to sleep after the procedure, and eye closure encourages proper corneal healing.[5] Steroidal and nonsteroidal anti-inflammatory agents, as well as an antibiotic, are instilled before and after surgery.[6,7] When selecting an antibi-

61

otic, gentamicin is sometimes avoided because of epithelial toxicity.[5] Although fluoroquinolones are not epitheliotoxic, the reported side effects of precipitates may have a questionable association with interface opacities.[5] Medications the patient normally takes can be continued; however, anticoagulants, such as aspirin, are avoided to reduce the risk of a subconjunctival hemorrhage.[6]

Preparing the Patient

When preparing the patient, he or she is given a cap to wear.[8] The lids are scrubbed to debride the lash area.[6] The other eye is covered to avoid cross-fixation of the fixation light.[9] Proparacaine is instilled for anesthesia.[6] Some surgeons prefer tetracaine or lidocaine.[5] The anesthesia is instilled immediately before the procedure to reduce epithelial toxicity.[5] Other surgeons like to instill anesthesia during preparation of the lids and draping, and again just before the keratectomy.[9] Sometimes pilocarpine is instilled to reduce discomfort due to microscope light glare.[5] Another reason for miosis is to make it easier to center the laser. The pupil center is used to avoid postoperative night glare.[5,10] However, some surgeons prefer to use the optic axis over the pupil center for centration.[8] Another variation is selecting the midpoint between the 2 axes (optic and pupillary), if there is a large angle kappa.[5]

In bilateral procedures, the second eye experiences a greater sensation during the procedure referred to as the *second eye syndrome*. The reasons for the sensation are unclear. One factor may be the patient's anticipation of the procedure. Another factor may be tachyphylaxis of the eye due to repeated proparacaine application.[5] While the patient is being prepared, the laser is programmed with the refractive data. For larger ablation zones, a deeper ablation is necessary.[8] Most procedures are multizone ablations, which are preferred over a single zone ablation.[11]

Thorough instructions are given to the patient to facilitate cooperation. The patient may feel some discomfort and blurring of vision as the procedure is performed. A feeling of pressure may result from the application of the suction ring. To ease his or her fears, the patient should also be familiarized with the sound of the excimer laser.

After a topical anesthetic is applied, povidone-iodine 7.5% (Betadine) is used to prepare the eyelids. A fenestrated, sterile, plastic, adhesive drape is placed. Some surgeons prefer not to use a drape because it may interfere with the path of the microkeratome and create flap complications. If a drape is not used, the eyelashes are cut or folded back with a Merocel surgical spear.[1] The drape keeps the eyelashes away from the operating field.[8] Meibum from the meibomian glands can cause interface opacities. Because the glands can be expressed by simple handling of the lids, the orifices should also be covered.[5,12]

An eye speculum is used to separate the eyelids.[1] Head positioning is very critical.[8] The head should be parallel to the floor, positioned with the chin and forehead in the same frontal plane.[2,13] Improper positioning can result in undesirable postprocedure refractive errors. The patient is instructed to remain as still as possible while fixating on the operating microscope's light.[8] For narrow or small palpebral fissures, obtaining adequate exposure can be problematic when making the cut. Turning the head away nasally shifts the eye temporally and allows better exposure. After the cut is made, the head is properly positioned for the ablation.[5] Use of powderless gloves is very important. Opacities result from the powder released from surgical gloves.[8] Interface opacities trapped under the flap is a well-documented complication of LASIK (see Chapter 8, LASIK Complications and Management).

Microkeratomes

The microkeratome is used to make the flap during the most difficult part of the procedure: the keratectomy. At the present time, the microkeratome mostly used is the Chiron's Automated Corneal Shaper of Ruiz.[6,14] Other microkeratomes are Storz's Draeger lamellar rotor microkeratome (semiautomatic), MicroPrecision's microkeratome (manual), Phoenix Keratek's Universal Keratome (automatic), Herbert Schwind Gimble and Co.'s Schwind Microkeratome (automatic), Moria's Moria/Plancon Microtech Lamellar Keratoplasty System (manual), LaserSight Technologies' Automatic Disposable Keratome (automatic), Hansa Research and Development's Hansatome (automatic), Eye Tech Ltd.'s Krumeich (automatic), TurboKeratome (SCMD) distributed by Microtech (manual), Eye Technology's Microlamellar Keratome (manual), Refractive Technologies' Flapmaker Disposable Microkeratome (automatic), and Clear Corneal Keratome of Guimaraes (manual).[8,15–17] Some surgeons prefer manual microkeratomes because they offer greater control. Other surgeons prefer the controlled speed of the automated microkeratomes.[8] On the horizon are nonmechanic keratomes featuring picosecond lasers and waterjet technologies (see Chapter 11, Future Techniques and Investigational Procedures).

Pearl:
LASIK is 90% keratectomy and 10% laser.[18]

The Hansatome microkeratome is different because it makes superior hinges instead of nasal hinges. The procedure is referred to as *down-up LASIK*. The cut is performed from the bottom of the cornea upward. The lid glides over the flap in a more natural way. The blink helps to smooth the flap. The patient is more comfortable because the foreign body sensation immediately after the procedure is reduced.[9] Another advantage is the very large flap created. The diameter is 9.5 to 10.0 mm instead of the average 8.5 mm with other microkeratomes. This enables a larger ablation zone to be made. The large flap offers greater moldability. With the larger flap size, microfolds formed in smaller flaps after the procedure are reduced.[8] Disadvantages of the Hansatome microkeratome are the surgeon cannot visualize the cut as it is performed, and the blade is not well-protected and can be easily damaged. Making a larger flap also has greater risk of cutting vessels that are located in the peripheral cornea.[9]

Setting up the microkeratome, and suction ring such as the one made by Chiron, requires over 30 steps of preparation.[19] Some surgeons prefer to perform the preflight check themselves rather than leaving it to an assistant.[12] The surgeon must make certain the microkeratome moves smoothly over the entire track without any obstructions.[1] For a bilateral procedure, use of a new blade (after careful examination) reduces flap complications.[1,3]

Pearl:
If there is any question about integrity of the microkeratome, sharpness of the blade, or operation of the microkeratome, do not proceed.[20]

Making the Cut

The cornea is marked to enable better repositioning of the flap at the end.[8] Accurate markings are needed to ensure proper alignment.[5] There are several markers available: Ruiz, Burrato, Chayet, Mendez, etc. The most popular is Ruiz, with an inner circle of 3 mm and outer circle of 10.5 mm joined by a pararadial segment.[13]

After the cornea is marked, a suction ring is applied (Figure 6.1).[5] The intraocular pressure is raised to ensure an optimum cut.[19] Loss of suction is very common, and the surgeon needs to be wary of it. It can result in a thin or irregular flap.[21] Applanation tonometry is performed to ensure the eye has a minimum pressure of 65 mm Hg.[8] A pressure in the range of 100 mm Hg is desirable.[5] At this point, the patient usually remarks that he or she cannot see.[13] When the pupil dilates after the application of the suction ring, the pressure should be correct; however, this is not always the case. The surgeon can recheck the pressure with finger pressures.[22]

The cornea is profusely irrigated with balanced salt solution while a suction tube removes the excess. The suction ring can be placed approximately 1 mm nasal (for a nasal hinge) to allow better centration of the treatment area and protect the hinge and undersurface of the flap from accidental ablation.[5,8] In case a short flap is made, ablation is still possible because of the nasal displacement.[1] It is best not to make a cut along any neovascularized areas of the cornea. The incision of vessels can cause bleeding and complicate the surgery. For conditions such as superficial limbal keratitis, the flap can be decentered inferiorly.[5] If performing a down-up procedure, the Hansatome is decentered superiorly.[2] The ring is placed toward the intended base of the flap.[8]

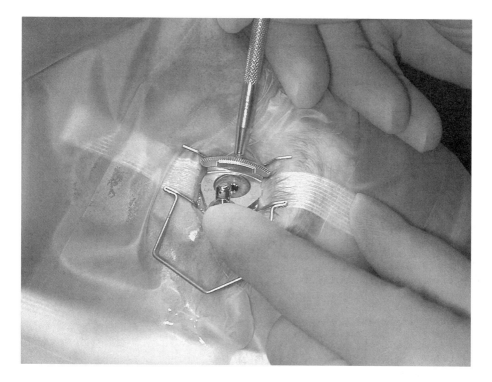

FIGURE 6.1. The eye is shown with the suction ring applied. (Courtesy of Steve Linn, OD, Hunkeler Eye Centers, Kansas City, MO.)

The flap varies with corneal curvature, corneal diameter, and suction pressure. The average is 8.5 mm in diameter, with a range of 7.2–9.0 mm.[5] Small diameter and steep corneas produce larger flaps.[5] An applanation lens can be used to predict the size and centration of the flap.[5]

Pearl:
Irrigation is necessary to prevent complications such as interface opacities. [8]

After moistening, the microkeratome is applied to the suction ring and the flap is made.[14] The keratome moves forward and then stops as the shaper hits the stop. The footswitch is depressed in the reverse position. If the flap does not return to the cornea during the reverse movement, then a cap instead of a flap may have been made. The surgeon needs to watch carefully if a cap is made.[8] Normally, a free cap can be found in the head of the microkeratome.[8]

Pearl:
Good flap quality results in easier and more comfortable retreatment.[1]

The suction ring is removed and the flap is lifted, leaving an exposed stromal bed. Before the flap is lifted, copious irrigation is again applied. Different instruments, such as a forceps or dry air cannula, can be used to lift the flap. The stromal side of the flap (the inside surface) is covered by a flap protector.[8]

Pearl:
A bad flap almost always means a bad operation.[12]

Flap thickness can be found with ultrasonic pachymetry. The flap thickness should be thick enough to prevent wrinkles, but thin enough to prevent the edge at the base from protruding and inducing irregular astigmatism.[8] A disadvantage of the thick flap is that less cornea is available for ablation. This may prove difficult for a high myope.[23] Flap thickness also affects outcomes. Two identical eyes would have different outcomes with different flap thicknesses. The ablation rates differ with each level of corneal stroma. This difference can affect the reliability and repeatability of the outcomes.[8]

Pearl:
Because different levels of corneal stroma have different ablation rates, the LASIK algorithm is difficult to standardize.[8]

Ablation

The amount of hydration in the stromal bed can also have a large effect on the outcome. In a myopic ablation, undercorrections and central islands may result. Some lasers compensate for hydration in their algorithms. Other lasers require pretreatment in the central 3 mm of the ablation area. This can be supplemented with using air or wiping with a surgical spear. The scanning excimer lasers do not require pretreatment.[5]

Ablation profiles are different between myopia and hyperopia. Myopic algorithms flatten the central cornea. Hyperopic profiles steepen the peripheral cornea. There are usually three zones described when dealing with hyperopic LASIK ablation patterns: total ablation diameter, blend zone, and optic zone. The total ablation diameter consists of the blend zone and optic zone. The blend zone is the transition zone outside of the optic zone.[24] One of the challenges of hyperopic LASIK is a small optic zone, resulting in glare and halo effects.[25]

The stroma is ablated. If there is no tracking system in the laser, the eye can be grasped by forceps to maintain position. A Thornton ring can also stabilize the eye.[8,14] Other surgeons use the suction ring to ensure proper positioning.[1] The ablation itself normally takes 30–60 seconds.[26] The interface is copiously irrigated to remove particles and epithelial cells.[14] For irregular surfaces, some surgeons pass a wet sponge with artificial tears over the ablation. This is followed by a 9 μm PlanoScan phototherapeutic keratectomy to smooth the surface.[8]

Replacing the Flap

The flap is repositioned by two techniques: dry and wet.[8] In the dry technique, the stromal bed is aspirated with a small suction tube to remove any debris or particles. The flap is folded back immediately to avoid exposing the stromal bed unnecessarily to foreign material.[27] The flap is replaced in a smooth, even motion to avoid complications.[5] With the wet technique, the ablated bed and stromal side of the flap are thoroughly flushed several times to remove debris. A Merocel microsponge is used to remove excessive moisture.[8]

The flap is repositioned with a cannula or spatula and adjusted with two microsponges.[4,8] The flap marks are used to properly align the cornea.[8] After the flap is repositioned, the interface is irrigated. The irrigation removes any interface debris and allows the flap to be floated back into position.[9] Floating the flap back into position is similar to plate tectonics. The earth's crust (the flap) moves on a bed (stromal bed) that is more fluid (irrigated).[12] The flap can be painted into alignment with the microsponges.[9] Once the flap is positioned, the gutter, or flap edge, is aspirated while still being irrigated. This ensures that debris at the flap edge are removed.[12] The corneal surface is then dried, because dehydration aids adhesion.[8] Some surgeons use a stream of oxygen for flap drying.[1,4] Others use a Merocel sponge.[1] Surgeons who prefer not to use air believe it may cause cracks in Bowman's membrane.[12] The flap edge is then repeatedly touched to dry the cornea.[1] It is checked for adhesion by depressing the peripheral host cornea and making certain the flap is also indented.[14] If the radiating lines extending from the peripheral cornea into the flap appear, the flap is adhering. The appearance of these lines into the flap is called the *striae sign* or the *Slade striae test.*[5,8] A microsponge can be used to lightly press the central cornea.[8] A gentle massage that stretches the flap in all directions helps to eliminate wrinkles. Pushing the edge of the flap to the edge of the bed also minimizes the peripheral scar and epithelial ingrowth.[25] When the flap is replaced, there is usually a gutter in the stromal bed surrounding the flap edge. The gutter is formed because the flap falls short of lining up with the original cut. The gutter must be kept dry to avoid central islands in the postablation phase.[28]

Pearl:
The surgeon must be able to manage fluids at all times, using the following techniques: cutting the wet cornea, maintaining even hydration during the ablation, and keeping the flap edge, or gutter, dry in the postablation phase. [2]

The cornea can be lightly sponged with diclofenac sodium (Voltaren), tobramycin-dexamethasone (Tobradex), and 1% cyclopentolate.[8] Some surgeons like to apply a bandage lens for protection.[1,8] Others prescribe a bandage lens only for epithelial defects.[3]

Pearl:
Avoidance of irregular astigmatism is the greatest challenge of lamellar surgery.[5,12]

Releasing the Patient

Postoperatively, a nonsteroidal anti-inflammatory agent and antibiotic steroid combination is instilled.[7] One common example is prescribing diclofenac (Voltaren) and dexamethasone (TobraDex) for 1 week. Nonpreserved artificial tears are prescribed up to every half hour for the first 48 hours after surgery.[6,29] The patient is instructed not to rub the operated eyes.[8] A slit-lamp evaluation is made to ensure the flap is in its place.[8] Some surgeons prefer to have the patient hold his or her eyes shut for 5 minutes and check the flap 15–30 minutes after the surgery.[5] Patients are released with a clear shield until the follow-up visit the next day. The shield largely protects the eye from displacement or tearing of the flap[1,6] (see Chapter 7, Postprocedure Management).

Retreatment

One major advantage of LASIK is the adjustability of the procedure. A surgeon can lift the flap years after the initial surgery for a retreatment or enhancement.[27]

In co-management, the patient is followed at regular intervals. Refractive error is monitored carefully. If the patient has an under- or overcorrection, another procedure can correct the residual. Because hyperopia, myopia, and astigmatism can be treated, enhancements are extremely worthwhile and viable. At the time of this writing, amounts as small as ± 0.50–0.75 D can be treated. Myopic enhancements can usually correct up to 2 D.

Two factors determine the time a retreatment should be performed: refractive stability and corneal wound healing.[30] Normally, the maximum postprocedure refractive changes occur in 1–3 months.[30] The maximum regression occurs between 2 and 4 weeks postprocedure.[23] Small changes in refraction follow. After 6 months, there is usually stability. The topographic maps and refractions should be consistent over a 2-week time period before the secondary surgery. On the other hand, the flap becomes more difficult to lift as time passes. Up to 9 months after the procedure, the flap can still be lifted.[30] However, some surgeons prefer to recut rather than lift the flap after 6 months.[23] After 1 year, lifting the flap is possible, but more difficult due to the healing process. An ideal time is 3–6 months after the initial procedure to ensure refractive stability and easier flap lifting.[30]

For patients with high myopia, there is a greater chance that retreatment is needed after the first procedure. Some surgeons tell all patients with 10 D or more of myopia that retreatment is required; however, the majority of patients do not need an enhancement.[23] The results of retreatments are highly favorable. One study shows that 98% of the retreated eyes were within one line of preoperative visual acuity.[23]

Pearl:
Retreatment is like golf. The first procedure gets the patient onto the green. The second procedure, retreatment, putts the ball into the hole.[23]

Retreatment follows essentially the same steps as the procedure itself. The flap edge can be marked with a surgical marker.[30] A Hockey knife can be used to scratch the epithelium over a small section of the original cut.[1] Other methods include using a Sinskey intraocular lens hook, Fine forceps, or the Suarez or the Machat spreader to break the interface.[23,30] Lifting the flap can be performed at the slit lamp, because it is sometimes easier than in the laser room.[31] Because the overlying epithelium is broken, there is risk for irregular astigmatism. The overlying epithelium at the edge can tear and does not have the microkeratome cut's sharp edge.[12] Just like the original procedure, the flap is folded back and the cornea is ablated. The amount of stromal adhesion varies with each patient. Greater amounts of time since the first procedure increase adhesion. Patients with aggressive wound-healing characteristics or patients with flap problems, such as stromal melt or haze, can also have stronger adherence.[23] After the flap is lifted, the interface is inspected for epithelium or debris. Any epithelium in the interface needs to be gently scraped with a surgical blade.[23] The stromal bed is ablated, and the flap is repositioned and dried.[30] The patient is followed up in the same manner as in the original procedure.

For 24 hours after the enhancement, patients can experience a discomfort due to the epithelial defects.[23] The discomfort can be avoided by making another microkeratome cut; however, the risks involved with making another cut are revisited. Because the cornea is flatter, there is also greater risk of a free cap than before. If a second cut is made, it is usually made thicker (200 µm) to avoid creating a free cap.[23] Retreatments with flap lifting are usually preferred because they are relatively safe and effective.[32]

References

1. Handzel A. How to Shorten the Learning Curve. In IG Pallikaris, DS Siganos (eds), LASIK. Thorofare, NJ: Slack, 1998;153–163.

2. Slade SG, Doane JF. Personal LASIK Technique. In JJ Machat, SG Slade, LE Probst (eds), The Art of LASIK (2nd ed). Thorofare, NJ: Slack, 1999;163–167.
3. Pallikaris IG, Siganos DS, Papadaki TG. Personal LASIK Technique. In JJ Machat, SG Slade, LE Probst (eds), The Art of LASIK (2nd ed). Thorofare, NJ: Slack, 1999;201–206.
4. Zaldivar R. Personal LASIK Technique. In JJ Machat, SG Slade, LE Probst (eds), The Art of LASIK (2nd ed). Thorofare, NJ: Slack, 1999;217–222.
5. Machat JJ, Probst LE. Personal LASIK Technique. In JJ Machat, SG Slade, LE Probst (eds), The Art of LASIK (2nd ed). Thorofare, NJ: Slack, 1999;141–161.
6. Lingua RW (ed). The Essentials of LASIK and Its Co-management. Brea, California: TLC Laser Center, 1997.
7. Pallikaris IG, Siganos DS. Laser in situ keratomileusis to treat myopia: early experience. J Cataract Refract Surg 1997;23:39–49.
8. Pallikaris IG, Siganos DS, Papadaki TG. The Procedure. In IG Pallikaris, DS Siganos (eds), LASIK. Thorofare, NJ: Slack, 1998;129–135.
9. Buratto L. Down-up LASIK with the Chiron Hansatome. In JJ Machat, SG Slade, LE Probst (eds), The Art of LASIK (2nd ed). Thorofare, NJ: Slack, 1999;95–107.
10. El Danasoruy MA, Waring GO, El Maghraby A, et al. Excimer laser in situ keratomileusis to correct compound myopic astigmatism. J Refractive Surg 1997;13:511–520.
11. Barraquer C. Laser In Situ Keratomileusis. In L Burrato, SF Brint (eds), LASIK: Principles and Techniques. Thorofare, NJ: Slack, 1998;215–223.
12. Kritzinger MS, Updegraff SA. Personal LASIK Technique. In JJ Machat, SG Slade, LE Probst (eds), The Art of LASIK (2nd ed). Thorofare, NJ: Slack, 1999;193–199.
13. Burratto L, Brint S, Ferrari M. LASIK techniques. In L Burrato, SF Brint (eds), LASIK: Principles and Techniques. Thorofare, NJ: Slack, 1998;73–112.
14. Perez-Santonja JJ, Bellot J, Claramonte P, et al. Laser in situ keratomileusis to correct high myopia. J Cataract Refract Surg 1997;23:372–385.
15. Arbelaez MC, Perez-Santonja JJ, Ishmail JL, et al. Automated Lamellar Keratoplasy (ALK) and Laser Assisted In Situ Keratomileusis (LASIK). In ON Serdarevic (ed), Refractive Surgery: Current Techniques and Management. New York: Igaku-Shoin, 1997;131–150.
16. Slade SG, Doane JF, Ruiz LA. Laser Myopic Keratomileusis. In DT Azar (ed), Refractive Surgery. Stamford, Conn: Appleton and Lange, 1997;357–365.
17. Doane J, Slade SG. Microkeratomes. In JJ Machat, SG Slade, LE Probst (eds), The Art of LASIK (2nd ed). Thorofare, NJ: Slack, 1999;79–94.
18. Machat JJ (ed). Excimer Laser Refractive Surgery: Practice and Principles. Thorofare, NJ: Slack, 1996.
19. Beran RF, Doty J. Laser Assisted In Situ Keratomileusis (LASIK). In RF Beran, J Doty (eds), The Surgical Management of Myopia and Astigmatism: a Guide for Optometrists. Columbus, OH: Anadem, 1996;87–101.
20. Casebeer JC. A systemized approach to LASIK. In L Burrato, SF Brint (eds), LASIK: Principles and Techniques. Thorofare, NJ: Slack, 1998;225–228.

21. Nataloni R. Hanastome reduces flap complications. Ocular Surg News 1998;16(14):37.
22. Singer HW. Ocular Surgery News International Edition. Jan 1998.
23. Probst LE, Machat JJ. LASIK Enhancement Techniques and Results. In JJ Machat, SG Slade, LE Probst (eds), The Art of LASIK (2nd ed). Thorofare, NJ: Slack, 1999;225–238.
24. Anschutz T, Pieger S. Evaluation of hyperopic photoablation profiles. J Refract Surg 1998;14:S192–S196.
25. Arbelaez MC. Hyperopic LASIK with the Chiron Technolas Excimer Laser. In JJ Machat, SG Slade, LE Probst (eds), The Art of LASIK (2nd ed). Thorofare, NJ: Slack, 1999;311–315.
26. Rama P, Chamon W, Genisi C, et al. Excimer Laser Intrastromal Seratomileusis (LASIK). In R Elander, LF Rich, JB Robin (eds), Principles and Practice of Refractive Surgery. Philadelphia: Saunders, 1997;455–469.
27. Waring GO. Future Developments in LASIK. In IG Pallikaris, DS Siganos (eds), LASIK. Thorofare, NJ: Slack, 1998;367–370.
28. Holliday J. Restoring stretch to Bowman's membrane reduces LASIK islands. Ocular Surg News 1997;15(11):14.
29. DePaolis M. Update on ocular surface protection rehabilitation. Primary Care Optom News 1997;12:1–15.
30. Salah T. Reoperation following LASIK. In IG Pallikaris, DS Siganos (eds), LASIK. Thorofare, NJ: Slack, 1998;305–315.
31. Siepser SB. A better technique may exist for lifting the flap in LASIK. Ocular Surgery News 1998;16(24):26.
32. Durrie DS. Aziz AA. Lift-flap retreatment after laser in-situ keratomileusis. J Refract Surg 1999;15:150–153.

CHAPTER 7

Postprocedure Management

Robert A. Ryan and Arthur B. Epstein

Few situations in the practice of eye care rival the sense of gratification achieved from guiding a patient through successful LASIK surgery. The arduous task of transforming a simple inquiry through the selection, education, and work-up process, into a well-prepared, keratorefractive surgical candidate has been described in great detail in the preceding chapters. The culmination of this complex process can often be appreciated during the follow-up period. When LASIK is executed properly, zealous patients often become the most loyal, gracious, exuberant source of new patient referrals to the practice. It is, however, imperative to familiarize oneself with Chapter 8, LASIK Complications and Management, as early detection and treatment are key to assuring satisfactory outcomes. Obviously, not all patients achieve ideal outcomes, and recognizing and dealing with such unanticipated problems are important aspects of skilled postoperative LASIK management.

Immediate Postoperative Period

As noted in Chapter 6, Description of Primary Procedure and Retreatment, topical anesthesia is achieved before initiating LASIK and is maintained throughout the procedure. The effect will likely persist for several minutes after completion of the procedure and undoubtedly keeps the patient comfortable in the immediate postoperative period. The greatest amount of discomfort in uncomplicated LASIK procedures occurs during the first 24 hours after surgery. Some patients will report burning and light sensitivity, and although not universal, this is quite normal. Many, if not all patients will be surprised by a dramatic improvement in their vision as they arise from the surgical table. This is especially true of mildly myopic patients who may achieve near 20/20 vision immediately after surgery.

All patients should be evaluated at the slit lamp 20–30 minutes after surgery for their response, as well as corneal flap position, regularity, and adherence (Figures 7.1 and 7.2). In most cases, the flap will be well-positioned with no folds or striae visible. In the event that this is not the case, corrective action, including repositioning or refloating and smoothing the flap, can and should be accomplished immediately.[1]

Postoperative Medications

As LASIK popularity has increased, there has been a growing number of reports of postoperative infections anecdotally and in the literature.[2-5] Although the exact mechanism of infection remains uncertain, the procedure clearly exposes the vulnerable stroma to endogenous bacteria. Most surgeons apply prophylactic topical antibiotic drops perioperatively. Although the effectiveness of this remains unproven, topical antibiotics reduce ocular surface bacterial loads and, theoretically, the risk of infection. Several commercially available antibiotics are commonly used; however, the fluoroquinolone class of drugs is probably the most common, as well as the more prudent because of the drugs' effectiveness, rapid kill rate, broad spectrum, and relatively low toxicity.

It is noteworthy that Binder and Hovding have challenged the indications for prophylactic antibiotic use. However, although the epithelium is essentially intact within hours after competent surgical treatment, most prudent providers recommend a short course (3–7 days) of a fluoroquinolone or an aminoglycoside t.i.d. or q.i.d. be continued postoperatively.[6,7] Tried-and-true aminoglycosides, such as tobramycin and gentamicin, are certainly reasonable choices due to their broad-spectrum efficacy against gram-

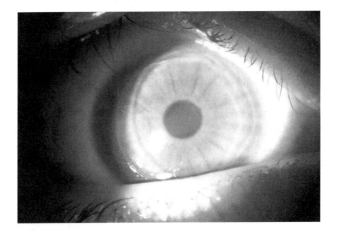

FIGURE 7.1. Immediate post-LASIK photograph. Note how apparent the temporal edge is due to epithelial gutter. Alignment markings are still apparent but will disappear within hours.

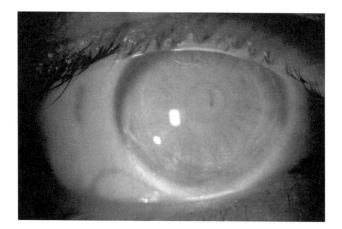

FIGURE 7.2. Immediate post-LASIK photograph. Appreciate the minimal NaFl staining even at flap margin.

negative bacteria and coverage against most gram-positive bacteria. The potential for epithelial toxicity, and associated delayed healing, may discourage their selection. However, this is rarely an issue for short-term, q.i.d. therapy of less than 1 week, such as would be anticipated for postoperative therapy.

Fluoroquinolone use (ciprofloxacin 0.3% [Ciloxan], manufactured by Alcon [Ft. Worth, TX], and ofloxacin 0.3% [Ocuflox], manufactured by Allergan [Irvine, CA]) is commonly used q.i.d. for 3–4 days or until epithelial closure, owing to the extremely efficacious profile of these agents with minimal associated toxicity. In addition, anti-inflammatory treatment is frequently recommended as standard postoperative protocol. Often, fluorometholone acetate 0.1% (Flarex), manufactured by Alcon, prednisolone acetate (Pred forte), manufactured by Allergan, or phosphate 0.1% (Inflamase Forte), manufactured by Ciba Vision (Duluth, GA), is prescribed q.i.d. to quiet stromal inflammation and edema, which actually may enhance healing rates. In contrast to the usual 4–7 day regimen after LASIK, patients who have PRK will generally be instructed to continue a topical steroid q.i.d. for 1–3 months with a slow taper over the next 2–4 months. This should be adjusted for each particular case, depending on the clinical findings. Those who display a more aggressive healing response, anterior stromal haze associated with marked regression, should increase dosing to perhaps every 1–2 hours for the next 4–6 weeks, with an ensuing slow taper over the next 4–6 months. Other individuals who appear overcorrected with a clear anterior stroma may have unusually poor healing characteristics. Immediate discontinuation of the steroid regimen should be suggested with careful follow-up to monitor for haze or regression. In this fashion, perhaps the refractive outcome can be modulated in some individuals.

Noninflammatory drops are frequently applied intraoperatively; however, their role is subject to debate.[8] Several rationales are offered for using anti-inflammatory medications. Nonspecific diffuse interface keratitis (or diffuse lamellar keratitis) is an inflammatory condition that infrequently occurs shortly after LASIK is performed.[9,10] Intraoperative stromal applications of topical steroids may decrease the incidence of diffuse lamellar keratitis.[11]

Many patients report discomfort or burning immediately after surgery. This is likely caused by trauma from the procedure, toxicity of the intraoperative medications, and the residual epithelial gutter defect at the edges of the flap. Topical nonsteroidal drops may minimize this initial discomfort and generally make the surgical experience more pleasant.

Many practitioners believe that topical steroids have little effect on the ultimate result and that their use has no scientific bearing. It would seem that this is indeed the case for many noncompliant patients we have treated. How to predict which patients may benefit from steroid therapy remains unknown. Prudent practitioners should elect to treat all patients and tailor modification to suit each particular patient based on the clinical response. The contrast from extended steroid use with PRK to very limited use after LASIK is believed to be due to physiologic differences in anterior and posterior stroma, as well as to changes in precorneal tear film chemistry after surface ablation. The anterior stroma is more populated with keratocytes than is evident histologically in the more posterior stroma. Keratocytes may be activated and transformed into fibroblasts as a result of excimer treatment. Also, inflammatory mediators are released into the tear film as a result of trauma to the delicate epithelium associated with PRK. Neither of these physiologic responses has been found to be a significant issue with LASIK surgery.

Nonsteroidal anti-inflammatory drugs (NSAIDs), such as ketorolac tromethamine 0.5% (Acular), manufactured by Allergan, and diclofenac sodium 0.1% (Voltaren), manufactured by Ciba Vision Ophthalmics, can effectively manage postoperative discomfort, and are especially indicated for pain management when epithelial defects are present. However, topical NSAIDs may delay epithelial healing and should be used with caution.[2] An increasing number of reports of corneal toxicity associated with the use of topical generic diclofenac sodium 0.1% have been noted.[12] Nonetheless, steroid and nonsteroid drops appear to be equally effective anti-inflammatory medications in LASIK patients.[13]

Lubrication in the postsurgical LASIK patient is of extreme importance. Dry eye is common, and various etiologies have been proposed. Whether severed corneal nerves, changes in surface topography, reduced eyelid apposition, or damaged goblet cell populations are responsible, dry eye symptoms seem to be the rule rather than the exception. Even asymptomatic patients appear to recover more rapidly with a well-hydrated ocular surface. A typical regimen includes copious lubrication with nonpreserved (or biocompatibly preserved) artificial tears (such as Refresh or Celluvisc manufactured by Allergan), perhaps as frequently as every hour. In the presence of epithelial defects, clinically observable signs of dry eye, and subjective complaints, lubrication should be even more frequent. Refractive procedures insult the corneal surface or, as is the case with LASIK, sever corneal nerves and decrease corneal sensitivity.[14] Intact surface innervation is a key requirement for maintenance of normal tear function and surface morphology.[15] In some patients, especially highly myopic or astigmatic patients associated with deeper ablations, more aggressive treatment may be needed, including temporary or semipermanent punctal plugs. Where appropriate, dry eye management should include warm compresses and lid hygiene to maintain healthy meibomian gland function, which will foster an effective evaporative barrier. White surface goblet cell density may be diminished by LASIK surgery and reports suggest that certain artificial-tear drops, such as TheraTears Advanced, may restore goblet cell levels.[16,17]

Postoperative Eye Protection: Protective Shields and Contact Lenses

Because displacement or damage to the flap is a primary concern, most surgeons suggest eye protection following LASIK. This may take several forms, the most common being clear plastic shields that are taped in place. In addition, patients are typically advised to avoid any eye manipulation or even forceful lid closure. The shields are used to prevent accidental eye rubbing during the critical first hours, when the flap is most easily dislodged, and for sleeping. Not all surgeons recommend or use them, whereas others have patients continue their use while sleeping for up to 1 week. Sunglasses help manage the photophobia that many patients experience in addition to providing a protective barrier, and most surgeons dispense them as part of the postoperative kit.

   Most often, bandage lenses are not used unless poor epithelial adherence is noted intraoperatively, which can predispose the patient to epithelial ingrowth. An intact epithelium is believed to be one of the forces that stabilizes the corneal flap and keeps it in proper position during stromal healing. Some surgeons believe that a bandage lens may be helpful in protecting the flap from the shearing forces of the eyelids and use a bandage lens routinely for up to 12 hours, or longer in certain cases. There are risks associated with bandage lens use, including infection, flap edema (see Chapter 10, Corneal Topography and Contact Lenses After LASIK), and dislodgement of the flap on lens removal.[18] Bandage lenses should be removed carefully, with sufficient lubrication applied to float the lens free of the underlying corneal flap. Prophylactic antibiotics used commensurately with the bandage lens can reduce the risk of infection.

Some surgeons approach lid immobilization rather simply. Hypoallergenic tape may be used to immobilize the eyelids. Under no circumstances should a pressure patch be applied to a freshly dissected cornea, due to the increased risk of creating striae or altering the flap position. Anxiolytics, sleeping aids, and analgesics may be prescribed to ease apprehension at the surgeon's discretion.

Day 1

Any practitioner who has managed PRK patients will immediately recognize the magic of LASIK on greeting his or her first patient the day after the LASIK procedure. We recall the intense pain many of our PRK patients described during the early phase three U.S. Food and Drug Administration clinical trials in 1990. Standard treatment included cycloplegia, topical antibiotics, topical steroids, and pressure patching, with a mandatory 6-month waiting period before the fellow eye was eligible for treatment. Typical visual acuity measured between 20/60 and 20/400 through a de-epithelialized, edematous cornea for the first 72 hours.

Practitioners can expect the majority of LASIK patients to report little (if any) discomfort, to experience good visual recovery in the range of 20/20 to 20/50, and to have rested well without incident. Patients who are hyperopic, highly myopic (over –9 D), or have significant astigmatism require deeper ablations and may initially report greater symptoms and slower visual recovery. If expectations have been properly managed, the majority of patients will be satisfied with their vision even at this early examination. Refraction can be attempted with variable results and endpoints. Patients may report night vision problems or visual difficulty in low or ambient light. This generally will resolve over several weeks to months.

Typically, the biomicroscopic evaluation at this point is rather unimpressive. In fact, it may be difficult (or impossible) to identify the flap margin, because epithelial cells have migrated to fill the gutter created by the passing microkeratome, and marginal fibrosis has not yet occurred. A small number of patients may still have a peripheral gutter surrounding the flap edge. If present, it should be symmetric and evenly spaced and will typically resolve within a day. Infrequently, epithelial defects are discovered and must be monitored due to increased risk of epithelial ingrowth and infection, as the barrier has been violated. Again, refrain from pressure patching, which may dislodge the flap or introduce striae. The decision may be made to simply tape the lids closed or place a bandage lens if necessary, but careful observation in 24 hours may be preferable. It is not unusual to note interfacial debris, such as lint, filaments, cosmetic products, or other foreign bodies, that have eluded the surgeon's detection due to limitations of the operating microscope. Occasionally, this debris may incite a mild, very focal infiltration that is self-limiting and not visually significant. Subsequent evaluations over the next several days provide convincing evidence that lifting the flap to irrigate the interface is rarely warranted.

The position and integrity of the flap are carefully evaluated at this visit. Significant striae or positioning anomalies should be addressed promptly by referring the patient to the surgeon for immediate correction. A slight amount of flap edema may still be noted; however, this is unusual and typically caused by excessive flap manipulation or hydration during a complicated or protracted procedure. Reassurance is perhaps our role of greatest importance to patients at this stage. Most are noticeably excited by their recovery, but filled with questions that anxiety prevented them from asking their surgeon. Reiteration of postoperative instructions should occur during this visit. Patients are reminded to adhere to prescribed medical therapy, which typically includes a 4-day course of a fluoroquinolone q.i.d.; prednisolone acetate 1% q.i.d.; and frequent, ongoing, lubrication therapy.

Ultraviolet radiation protection is strongly encouraged to avoid fibroblast activation and induction of aggressive healing responses, which have been reported as much as 6 months after keratorefractive procedures.[19] Patients should be instructed to avoid visually intense tasks, strenuous exercise, swimming or hot tubs, heavy cleaning, and dirty environments for the next 4 days or until further notice. They should also be reminded of the importance of abstaining from rubbing their eyes. Written instructions are beneficial to enhance patient retention and compliance, and must include a means of contacting the practitioner on call should problems or questions arise.

One Week

At 1 week after LASIK, patients have generally returned to a normal daily routine, with all previous restrictions lifted, and are realizing the incredible benefits of having undergone corrective surgery. Many will report mildly fluctuating vision, difficulty driving at night or in dim illumination, and persistent dryness. Explaining that the flap is not fully healed, and that the tear chemistry and flow have been altered by the treatment and medication, will help individuals understand that these reactions are anticipated. Postoperative medications should have been discontinued for the past few days, and it is no longer necessary to use eye shields while sleeping. Ultraviolet protection and lubrication therapy should continue to be used for several months.

Unaided acuity is likely stable by now, and refraction should be performed. This will provide a benchmark to monitor for regression, and will reveal best corrected acuity, which, ideally, should equal or exceed presurgical levels. Any loss of best corrected acuity must be explained, as early intervention and correction are vital to successful outcomes. Fluorescein dye may highlight striae in the flap, although retroillumination through a large pupil fully enhances detection (Figure 7.3).[20] Frequently, interfacial debris is noted and is generally of little consequence (Figure 7.4). Videokeratoscopy may be performed, particularly if a complication is suspected or the visual outcome and/or best corrected visual acuity is less than expected. Color Plate 2 displays a corneal topographic map 1 week after LASIK, which reveals a central island, one reason that a patient's best corrected visual acuity may be decreased at this point in the postoperative period. Corneal topography generally provides more reliable and clinically useful data later in the postoperative course (see Chapter 10, Corneal Topography and Contact Lenses after LASIK).

Tonometry is suggested at this visit, but only after disclosure dyes have been used to determine epithelial integrity. Ideally, a Tono-Pen (XOMED Surgical Products, Boston, MA) or Pneumatonometer (Pneumatonometer Digilab, Boston, MA) should be used because it reduces the likelihood of flap displacement. Artificially low pressures, which vary with the amount of surgical correction, are common with Goldman and noncontact tonometry due largely to decreased corneal thickness.[21]

It is generally accepted that soft contact lens wear may be safely initiated by 1 month postoperatively. Situations that may merit lens use

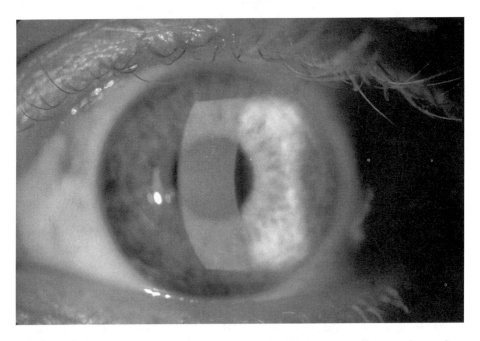

FIGURE 7.3. One week post-LASIK photograph. Observe visually significant fine striae within visual axis, enhanced by NaFl, and more obvious with retroillumination.

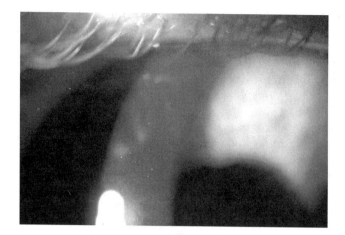

FIGURE 7.4. Refractile interfacial debris barely apparent at 1 week post-LASIK. Note lack of inflammatory response.

include overcorrection, undercorrection, and regression, as well as for demonstration of proposed outcomes (e.g., monovision, planned undercorrection for latent hyperopes or emerging presbyopes). In the rare instance in which contact lens correction is necessary, it is imperative to properly educate the patient to minimize flap insult. For patients with demonstrable dry eyes, it is reasonable to consider punctal occlusion where indicated, informing patients this reversible procedure may be beneficial indefinitely.

For some patients having difficulty with glare and night driving, an aberration-blocking soft contact lens may be helpful. Aspheric lenses using the panofocal effect, such as Specialty Choice AB (Specialty Ultravision, Campbell, CA) or Frequency 55 Aspheric (Cooper Vision, Irvine, CA), can help mitigate glare and improve contrast sensitivity. Success has been variable.

One Month

The primary goal of the 1-month visit is to measure visual acuity and refractive status for comparison to earlier findings. Scanning- and flying-spot technology laser treatments tend to stabilize sooner than their broad-beam counterparts, due to smoother transition zones and marginal blending. Again, patients may remark about fluctuations in subjective acuity due to the aforementioned reasons, but objective data are used to determine whether true change is present. It is also important to recognize the novelty of the improvement may wane, and patients may become more critical of their outcome over the first several weeks. If symptoms of flare or night vision problems were noted, they will likely have diminished or abated over the first month.

Pearl:
Patients may be more critical about their vision at the 1-month visit, because the novelty of their improvement may have worn off.

If epithelial ingrowth is to occur, it should be apparent by the 1-month visit. It is important to make careful record of this situation and measure its extent. Concern should be raised if cells invade the flap interface for greater than 1 mm from the margin, cause rolled or eroded flap margins, interfere with complete re-epithelialization, or lead to discomfort. Extensive ingrowth can encourage irregular astigmatism and limit the accuracy of the refractive data. Topographic measurements are expected to be reliable by this stage and can assist in diagnosing the etiology of less-than-ideal outcomes. For example, Figure 7.5 displays a clinically normal post-LASIK eye on slit lamp examination, but the topographic map displays a decentered ablation and irregularity at the flap edge, resulting in irregular astigmatism and a decrease in best corrected visual acuity.

Pearl:
Epithelial ingrowth will be evident by the 1-month visit.

At 1 month, careful refraction should be performed to determine refractive state and as a further baseline to access future regression. Auto-

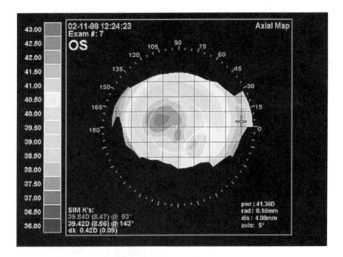

FIGURE 7.5. Decentered ablation and irregular astigmatism noted on an axial map after LASIK.

mated refraction may not be reliable after LASIK surgery, and caution should be used in relying on these measurements.[22] Overcorrections may be treated with topical NSAIDs using q.i.d. dosing. It has been observed that NSAIDs either stimulate epithelial remodeling or stromal fibroblast activity and appear to cause regression. Undercorrection should not be addressed unless the patient is highly disturbed and his or her initial correction was relatively low. The more myopic the patient initially, the greater the amount of time that should be allowed for stabilization before enhancement is undertaken.

Intermediate-Term Care

A reasonable follow-up schedule should include visits at 3, 6, and 12 months after surgery. Enhancements for all patients can often be entertained by the 3-month evaluation, providing the data are stable on refraction (cycloplegic preferred) and topography. There must be sufficient regression to warrant the risk of enhancement, and also enough treatment required to allow the surgical algorithm to blend adequately over the entire ablation zone. The criterion is typically a minimum of 1.00 D, or worse than 20/40 acuity. Some suggest deferring retreatment until additional measurements confirm stability over a longer period, but most experienced surgeons are comfortable intervening as early as 6 to 16 weeks after surgery. Another consideration in making the decision when to enhance is dependent on the patient's ability to function in the interim. In addition, one should scrutinize the flap margin for signs of fibrosis, which indicates flap healing (Figure 7.6).[23] The fibrosis marks the area of penetration through Bowman's membrane, and its size may be related to the immediate postoperative gutter. Most individuals can have the flap margin identified with a spatula and lifted with nontoothed forceps within 6 months of the surgical date. This reduces the risk associated with the primary procedure, as the microkeratome is not required in these cases. If a greater amount of time elapses or substantial marginal fibrosis is noted, the surgical plan may require another lamellar keratectomy, which increases intraoperative risk.

If regression is to occur, it is likely a function of combined etiologies. Certainly, the magnitude of the primary treatment relates to anticipated regression, due to remodeling during postoperative healing. In addition, healing characteristics vary among individuals. More aggressive healing, generally considered to affect less than 10% of the population domestically, is consistent with a greater degree of regression. Enhancement candidates are universally scheduled for a fraction of the correction attempted initially, and they are therefore much less likely to experience as significant a regression after retreatment. The importance of cycloplegic refraction cannot be overstated. Accommodative function can remain even in the presbyopic population and can substantially alter outcomes. Overcorrection is less desirable

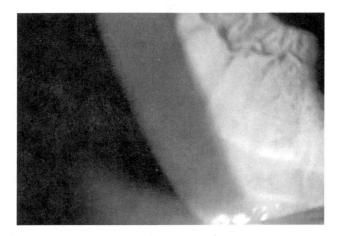

FIGURE 7.6. Early marginal fibrosis outlining flap edge 6 months post-LASIK.

than a slight undercorrection, as even impending presbyopes will often be device dependent. It is helpful to reassess the acceptance of undercorrection or monovision when appropriate because postoperative patients have now experienced a different refractive status and may respond more favorably.

Regression, when it occurs, can be expressed in terms of a percentage of the planned treatment. Regression appears to affect those with greater levels of myopia more frequently and to a greater magnitude. A patient with 10.00 D of myopia should expect a higher likelihood of regression than a patient with 2.00 D of myopia. Simply stated, if regression occurs, it is likely to result in more residual myopia for the individual who had greater refractive error preoperatively. As discussed in the section Intermediate-Term Care, regression must be substantial enough to warrant the risk of retreatment. One can therefore deduce that a patient with a higher level of ametropia should anticipate an increased chance of requiring multiple procedures to achieve the desired outcome.

For example, assume a patient with 10.00 D of myopia had LASIK performed and was found to have 20/20 acuity with no residual refractive error at 1 week after surgery. On re-evaluation 5 weeks later, acuity was reduced to 20/80 and –1.50 D restores 20/20 after cycloplegia. This represents a 15% regression from the initial treatment plan of –10.00 D. This particular patient was found to be stable over the next 6 weeks and was scheduled for enhancement for 1.50 D of residual myopia accordingly. Obviously, the surgical algorithm varies predicated on the refractive error correction desired (i.e., less stromal tissue ablated for lower levels of myopia treatment), which clinically appears to be associated with less regression.

Still, if we anticipate a 15% regression after the enhancement of –1.50 D, this individual will have approximately –0.25 D residual refractive error

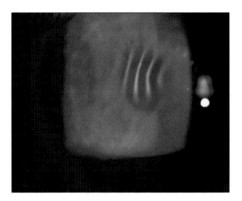

Color Plate 1. Full thickness corneal folds in a soft lens wearer clearly demonstrate the power of a soft lens to mold the cornea.

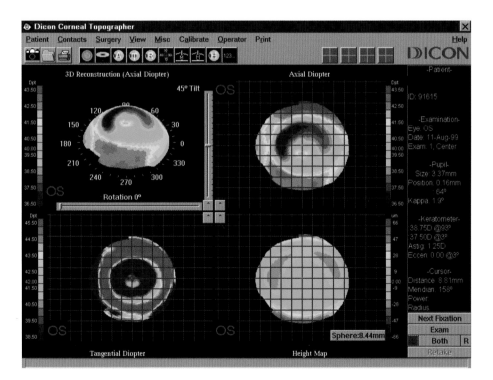

Color Plate 2. Central island noted after LASIK. The tangential diopter map best highlights the corneal irregularity, although the axial and 3D topographic displays can detect the central island.

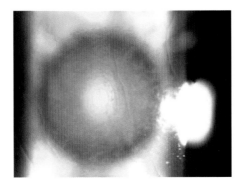

Color Plate 3. Picture of flap wrinkles.

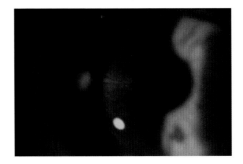

Color Plate 4. Encroaching epithelial ingrowth.

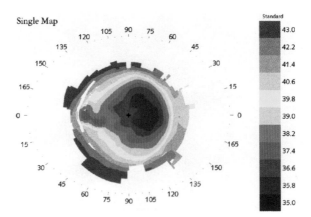

Color Plate 5. Topography of irregular astigmatism resulting from epithelial ingrowth raising flap edge.

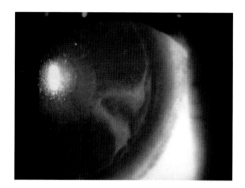

Color Plate 6. Flap thinning and corneal melt caused by epithelial ingrowth.

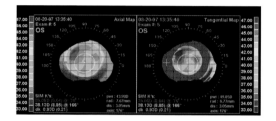

Color Plate 7. Post-ALK (automated lamellar keratoplasty) cornea imaged by the axial and instantaneous (tangential map) reconstruction algorithms. Note the cursor positioned over the same location on each map reads values that differ by almost 6 D. (Reprinted with permission from LB Szczotka, M Aronsky. Contact lenses after LASIK. J Am Optom Assoc 1998;69[12]:775–84.)

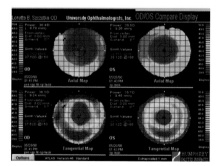

Color Plate 8. Post-LASIK corneas imaged by the axial and instantaneous (tangential) reconstruction algorithms. Note the axial maps image a central flat zone and the instantaneous maps image a smaller central flat zone with a very steep transitional ring. (Reprinted with permission from LB Szczotka, M Aronsky. Contact lenses after LASIK. J Am Optom Assoc 1998;69[12]:775–84.)

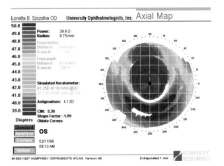

Color Plate 9. Post-LASIK topography with irregularity surrounding the flap. (Reprinted with permission from LB Szczotka, M Aronsky. Contact lenses after LASIK. J Am Optom Assoc 1998;69[12]:775–84.)

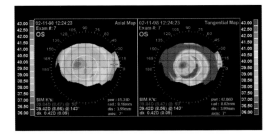

Color Plate 10. Postoperative LASIK patient with persistent hyperopic irregular astigmatism and a best corrected spectacle acuity of 20/80, 3 months after surgery. The same raw data are imaged by the axial and instantaneous (tangential) reconstruction algorithms. Note the cursor is positioned over the center of the "knee" of the transition zone on the axial map. (Reprinted with permission from LB Szczotka, M Aronsky. Contact lenses after LASIK. J Am Optom Assoc 1998;69[12]:775–84.)

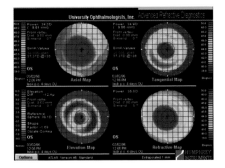

Color Plate 11. Four map view of a post-LASIK cornea. The elevation map presents relative heights above or below a reference sphere and does not represent curvature.

as a result of the healing response after the second procedure, as compared to –1.50 D of ametropic change after the initial treatment. As was stated in the section One Month, enhancements are preferred before the 6-month target to minimize the probability of substantial healing, which would require a fresh lamellar keratectomy. It is for these reasons that a conservative surgical approach is common, to ablate only the necessary amount of tissue to reach the desired outcome.

Addressing Unhappy Patients

Not every LASIK patient has an ideal outcome; some patients are dissatisfied with the results. Complications have been estimated to be between 3% and 5%, and this does not include a significant number of patients who experience mild, but noticeable, impairment. Clearly, the rate of complications vary with surgical skills and experience. Visual acuity is not always an accurate measure of visual performance. It is important to recognize this and to take patient complaints seriously, even in the face of apparent 20/20 acuity. Real-world performance is far more important to patients than objective findings. Doctors should validate patient complaints by listening and reassuring. This establishes a nonadversarial relationship in which problems can be solved.

In some situations, patients may believe that their surgical outcomes are so poor and dysfunctional that they regret their decision to have LASIK. Although dealing with such patients can be difficult, it is important to listen, and, when possible, try to address their complaints. In some cases, time will minimize these problems. Although it is important to remind patients of this and to reassure them, the line between being reassuring and patronizing can be a fine one.

Contact lenses may be helpful in treating these patients, but proper patient selection and expectation management are the best ways to prevent such problems from occurring. New topographically linked custom ablation surgical procedures may also be of value in retreatment or in future initial treatments.

References

1. Probst LE, Machat J. Removal of flap striae following laser in situ keratomileusis. J Cataract Refract Surg 1998;24:153–155.
2. Lam DS, Leung AT, Wu JT, et al. Culture-negative ulcerative keratitis after laser in situ keratomileusis. J Cataract Refract Surg 1999;25:1004–1008.
3. Mulhern MG, Condon PI, O'Keefe M. Endophthalmitis after astigmatic myopic laser in situ keratomileusis. J Cataract Refract Surg 1997;23:948–950.
4. al-Reefy M. Bacterial keratitis following laser in situ keratomileusis for hyperopia. J Refract Surg 1999;15:216–217.

5. Webber SK, Lawless MA, Sutton GL, Rogers CM. Staphylococcal infection under a LASIK flap. Cornea 1999;18:361–365.

6. Binder P, Worthen D. A continuous wear hydrophilic lens. Arch Ophthalmology 1976;94:2109–2111.

7. Hovding G. Conjunctival and contact lens bacterial flora during lens wear. Acta Ophth 1982;60:439–448.

8. Hersh P, Rice B, Baer J, et al. Topical nonsteroidal agents and corneal wound healing. Arch Ophthalmology 1990;108:577–583.

9. Kaufman SC, Maitchouk DY, Chiou AG, Beuerman RW. Interface inflammation after laser in situ keratomileusis. Sands of the Sahara syndrome. J Cataract Refract Surg 1998;24:1589–1593.

10. Smith RJ, Maloney RK. Diffuse lamellar keratitis. A new syndrome in lamellar refractive surgery. Ophthalmology 1998;105:1721–1726.

11. Peters NT, Lingua RW, Kim CH. Topical intrastromal steroid during laser in situ keratomileusis to retard interface keratitis. J Cataract Refract Surg 1999;25:1437–1440.

12. Alcon recalls its generic diclofenac. Primary Care Optometry News Nov 1999;4(11):10.

13. Vantesone DL, Luna JD, Muino JC, Juarez CP. Effects of topical diclofenac and prednisolone eyedrops in laser in situ keratomileusis patients. J Cataract Refract Surg 1999;25:836–841.

14. Kim WS, Kim JS. Change in corneal sensitivity following laser in situ keratomileusis. J Cataract Refract Surg 1999;25:368–373.

15. Tseng SC, Tsubota K. Important concepts for treating ocular surface and tear disorders. Am J Ophthalmol 1997;124:825–835.

16. Lenton LM, Albietz JM. Effect of carmellose-based artificial tears on the ocular surface in eyes after laser in situ keratomileusis. J Refract Surg 1999;15: S227–S231.

17. Gilbard J, Rossi S. An electrolyte-based solution that increases corneal glycogen and conjunctival goblet cell density in a rabbit model for keratoconjunctivitis sicca. Ophthalmology 1992;99:600–604.

18. Detorakis ET, Siganos DS, Houlakis VM, et al. Microbiological examination of bandage soft contact lenses used in laser refractive surgery. J Refract Surg 1998;14:631–635.

19. Nuss RC, Puliafito CA, Dehm E. Unscheduled DNA synthesis following excimer laser ablation of the cornea in vivo. Invest Ophthalmol Vis Sci 1987;28:287–294.

20. Rabinowitz Y, Rasheed K. Fluorescein test for the detection of striae in the corneal flap after laser in situ keratomileusis. Am J Ophthamol 1999;127:717–718.

21. Chatterjee A, Shah S, Bessant D, et al. Reduction in intraocular pressure after excimer laser photorefractive keratectomy. Ophthalmology 1997;104:355–359.

22. Salchow DJ, Zirm ME, Stieldorf C, Parisi A. Comparison of objective and subjective refraction before and after laser in situ keratomileusis. J Cataract Refract Surg 1999;25:827–835.

23. Machat J (ed). Excimer Laser Refractive Surgery: Practice and Principles. Thorofare, NJ: Slack, 1996.

CHAPTER 8

LASIK Complications and Management

Paul M. Karpecki and Steven H. Linn

LASIK has recently surpassed cataract surgery as the most common eye surgery performed in the world. As the main procedure for refractive surgery, LASIK co-management should be a well-established component of any optometric practice. The success of LASIK is driven largely by the accuracy of visual outcome, but also by patient comfort and rapid visual recovery. Because of these patient-driven factors, LASIK will be used for refractive vision correction for many years. New advances in lasers and microkeratomes will also drive LASIK to higher levels of accuracy and safety.

This chapter helps the optometrist to understand complications related to LASIK and to resolve concerns about normal and abnormal findings. Observing LASIK in the operating room is an important key to understanding co-management and complications; most surgeons welcome comanaging physicians into their operating rooms. Another important key is witnessing patients at different stages of their postoperative care.

Pearl:
Observing the LASIK procedure in the operating room is an important key to understanding co-management and complications.

Explanation of Procedure

LASIK begins with the application of a suction ring, which brings the globe to a taut 100+ mm Hg. An oscillating microkeratome is used to construct a hinged flap 160–180 μm in thickness. After the microkeratome and suction ring are removed, the flap is gently laid back to expose the stromal bed. The eye is then aligned and ablated with a predefined quantity of excimer laser energy. The flap is then repositioned, smoothed, and allowed to dry. The drying enhances the flap adherence before the eye is finally lubricated.

Complications are divided into three categories. The first, intraoperative complications, is usually associated with improper performance of devices or technique. The second, early postoperative complications, can be attributed to poor patient compliance or residual problems from the surgery. The third, late postoperative complications, is mostly due to individual patient healing differences. A list of common postoperative complications are listed in Table 8.1.

Intraoperative Complications and Treatment

Each microkeratome design brings to the procedure both common and unique risks. When certain types of microkeratomes are incompletely or incorrectly assembled (e.g., plate depths set too deep), perforation of the eye with loss of intraocular contents has been reported. This problem can be eliminated with newer designs of microkeratomes. If a microkeratome sticks or loses power, an incomplete flap may be created. The flap should be repositioned and allowed to heal for a minimum of 3 months before the procedure is attempted a second time. If there is not enough cornea presenting through the suction ring, or if the microkeratome continues past the stop point, a free cap may result. It may be possible to continue with the procedure based on the size of stromal bed and anticipated ablation size. With the help of preoperative corneal markings, the cap can be repositioned and extra caution taken to make sure the cap is not displaced. If suction is lost or diminished, or if it fluctuates during passage of the microkeratome, the cut may be too thin, irregular, or donut-shaped (buttonhole). The blade may break through the epithelium in the center of the cornea and then return to the stroma, creating a donut-shaped flap. In these cases, the irregular flap should be returned to its original position without laser treatment. After 3 months of healing, allowing for refractive and topographic stability, the procedure can be repeated in most cases. Other postoperative flap complications are discussed in the section Early Postoperative Complications and Treatment.

TABLE 8.1
Complications from Various Studies

Complication	Frequency (%)	Study
Intraoperative flap complications	2.7%	Wilson[3]
Postoperative flap complications	4%	Wilson[3]
Epithelial ingrowth	14.7%	Wilson,[3] 4.3% Farah[4]
Epithelial ingrowth requiring removal	1.7%	Wilson[3]
Epithelial defects	5%	Davidorf[5]
Interface debris	6.8%	Farah[4]
Flap wrinkles	5.9%	Farah[4]

Once the flap is created and the stroma exposed, it is important for the surgeon to center the ablation on the cornea. This is usually done by having the patient fixate on a target within the housing of the delivery scope; the surgeon then centers the microscope reticule over the desired treatment area. The ablation could be decentered if the patient loses fixation or moves his or her head. This could lead to an unfavorable visual outcome with irregular astigmatism and loss of best corrected vision. Newer lasers incorporate efficient eye-tracking mechanisms that greatly reduce the incidents of decentered ablations.

Early Postoperative Complications and Treatment

Postoperative flap complications include the following: flap displacement, flap wrinkles, and folds. These complications most commonly occur in the first 24 hours after LASIK, before the epithelium has had time to heal over the lamellar entry site. Early complications may be owing to several reasons: a surgeon's not allowing enough time for the flap to dry and adhere to the bed, a patient's manipulating his or her eye, or a patient's tight lids or proptotic eyes. To avoid early complications, the patient is instructed and given clear protective shields to wear while sleeping. The shields prevent any inadvertent pressure on the eye and keep the patient from rubbing his or her eye.

At the 1-day postoperative visit, if a flap is observed to have moved or developed folds or wrinkles, the surgeon is to be notified immediately so the flap can be refloated and positioned properly (Figure 8.1).

Folds or wrinkles (Color Plate 3) are not to be confused with Bowman's crinkles or microstriae. Patients with moderate to high refractive

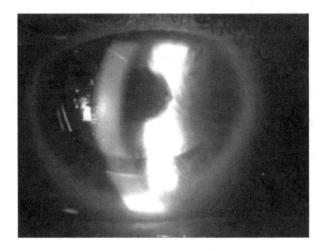

FIGURE 8.1. Picture of flap displacement.

errors present with these fine, vertical or horizontal, gray lines. These microscopic crinkles or microstriae in Bowman's layer are due to the anatomic disparity between the stromal bed and the flap after tissue has been removed. The condition may also be observed when excess irrigation and overhydration occur during the procedure.

An epithelial defect is an occurrence that usually appears near the flap edge because although all complications are rare, this is less rare than others. Due to the microkeratome suction ring and the manipulation of the flap, a patch of epithelium may slough off. If the patient has loose epithelium preoperatively, a defect is more likely to occur. Loose epithelium during surgery may be associated with recent contact lens use in some patients. An epithelial defect can best be managed with preservative-free artificial tears during the day and a thicker lubricating drop at bedtime. In rare occasions, when the patient is very uncomfortable and the lid is rubbing too abruptly over the defect, a bandage contact lens, such as an extended-wear disposable lens, may be used until the area is re-epithelialized. Until the epithelium is intact, the patient should be seen every day, postoperative antibiotics should be continued, and steroids should be discontinued. Remember to generously lubricate the eye before removing the lens by first sliding it to the conjunctiva.

Infection is a possible complication of any surgery. However, infection is very uncommon in LASIK, due to the more effective antibiotics used postoperatively and the proper sterile technique used during the procedure. Most refractive surgeons or optometrists will never see infection. An infection may be evident at the patient's first postoperative visit, 24 hours later, or it may occur 1–3 days after surgery. Postoperative instructions should include explaining the signs and symptoms of a possible infection. If the patient experiences an increase in blurry vision, redness, pain, or discharge, he or she should be advised to have an emergency examination.

Scattered debris at the interface level are common, and because they are generally inert, they will not create complications or affect the vision outcome. Debris at the interface bother the doctor, but not the patient. Sometimes, microcystic edema or infiltration of white blood cells may be noted around the debris and may cause some temporary visual disturbances. In these situations, low doses of steroids are recommended.

Diffuse lamellar keratitis (DLK), also known as the *sands of the Sahara*, is a noninfectious diffuse inflammation at the level of the interface. It appears similar to haze observed after photorefractive keratectomy. Anterior chamber reaction may or may not accompany DLK, or it may be the presenting sign. DLK is usually apparent within the first 1–7 days after surgery (Figure 8.2). The patient's presenting symptoms may include pain, photophobia, redness, and tearing. Current theories suggest that the etiology may be an immune response secondary to oils present in the microkeratome, excessive debris, dead bacterial particulate matter or exotoxins, thermal insult, or environmental humidity and temperature.

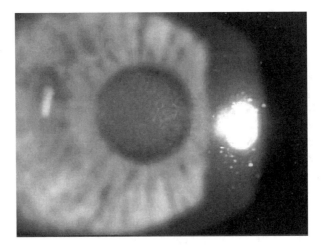

FIGURE 8.2. Picture of diffuse lamellar keratitis.

In the late 1990s, use of a desktop sterilization unit has been implicated as one of the causes of DLK. Despite following the manufacturer's recommendations for cleaning the unit, culture-positive *Pseudomonas* was found in the reservoir of the sterilization unit. Instituting a new regimen of draining the reservoir nightly, leaving it to dry overnight, and refilling it with sterile water the next day seems to alleviate the problem.

Cases of DLK should be treated with the following regimen: ofloxacin (Ocuflox), 0.3%, every 2 hours and prednisolone acetate (Pred Forte), 1%, every two hours, with cyclopentolate (Cyclogyl), 1%, added three times a day if significant photophobia is present for the first 24 hours. At the next-day visit, if the condition has improved, discontinue the cyclopentolate, and reduce the drops to four times a day. After the visit, continue to see the patient every few days until resolution, and then discontinue medication. If the inflammation has worsened and clumps of cells are seen aggregating centrally, the patient should be referred to the surgeon for prompt irrigation under the flap. Also, moderate to severe cases of DLK may require oral prednisolone (40–80 mg per day for 1 week) and/or lifting the flap and irrigating the interface as early as possible.

Late Postoperative Complications and Treatment

Central islands are defined as a central steepening greater than 1.5 D covering a 1.5-mm area, seen postoperatively after 1 month. Classic symptoms are ghosting or monocular diplopia. The surgeon may retreat these areas after 3 months with 30 pulses within a 2.5-mm zone. With new pretreatment software, central islands have virtually disappeared.

Epithelial ingrowth is most commonly detected at the 1-month visit. It appears as white, milky deposits at the level of the interface and should be carefully observed; it can become an aggressive ingrowth complication. Ingrowth should only be treated if one of the three following presentations exists:

1. Ingrowth obstructs the visual axis.
2. Ingrowth may not be in the visual axis, but it can cause irregular astigmatism (Color Plates 4 and 5).
3. Ingrowth is progressive and can lead to a corneal melt (Color Plate 6).

These presentations require returning to the surgery center to remove the ingrowth. Any epithelial ingrowth that appears to progress, or causes loss of overlying tissue or a drop in best corrected vision, requires referral to the surgery center. One study of 1,013 eyes that had LASIK reported that 14.7% had epithelial ingrowth, but only 1.7% required surgical intervention.

Progressive corneal ectasia is a complication that is becoming more prevalent internationally in high myopes. It appears as a progressive myopia or ectatic condition thought to be caused by weakened corneal tissue or not maintaining 250 μm of tissue under the flap after ablation. To avoid progressive corneal ectasia, pachymetry for high myopes is essential. Many of these patients may have to have a partial lamellar keratoplasty or full-thickness penetrating keratoplasty if the ectasia becomes advanced. With myopes who are 10 D or higher, it is wise to inform them they may not be candidates for LASIK until their corneal thickness is assessed.

Side Bar: Parameters to keep in mind before LASIK and enhancements include the following:

Average corneal thickness is 550 mm.
Microkeratome creates a 160-mm flap.
The corneal thickness that must remain under the flap for safety is 250 mm.
The excimer laser removes approximately 12 mm of tissue for each D of correction.
These parameters are especially important for high myopes above 10 D. Their corneal thickness may not be adequate to safely perform the procedure or an enhancement. The sum of the flap thickness (160 μm), the minimum stromal bed thickness (250 μm), and the attempted tissue removal (12 μm × D of correction) must all equal less than the patient's most recent central corneal pachymetry measurements.

Irregular astigmatism and associated loss of best spectacle-corrected visual acuity are two of the most common complications of LASIK.[1] Causes include irregular flap cuts, flap misalignment, epithelial ingrowth, irregularities of laser ablation due to decentration, and resulting central islands. Another factor contributing to irregular astigmatism is the small amount of disparity between the bed and the posterior surface of the flap. These problems are not easily resolved, and, if extensive, patients may need to wait until technology brings such solutions as topography-guided ablations or ablatable gel masks (see Chapter 11, Future Techniques and Investigational Procedures). In the meantime, adequate consultation with the surgeon and patient reassurance are important.

Regression of effect, overcorrection, undercorrection, and regular astigmatism can be temporarily treated with spectacle correction until adequate refractive stabilization. Most surgeons feel comfortable with retreating these conditions after the 3-month visit.

Side Bar: Early postoperative refractive errors.

During the first month, the patient's refractive error most likely will be slightly overcorrected. This is due to the calculated laser nomograms, which anticipate a natural regression of effect. Induced astigmatism may also be detected because of corneal remolding or tear film disruption. These are normal early healing symptoms and should not be confused with complications.

Careful consideration regarding enhancements is necessary at the 3-month visit. Many patients are happy with their vision regardless of the result. As clinicians, we should base our decisions on whether the patient is 20/happy or 20/unhappy. As concerned practitioners, we tend to place our expectations on the patient and often convince them that retreatment is necessary. Remember to treat the patient, not the refraction. Most patients do not wish to have further surgical procedures. Certainly, any borderline cases can be referred to the surgeon for retreatment evaluation.

Guidelines used for retreatment at Hunkeler Eye Centers in Kansas City include the following:

- Refractive error greater than or equal to 0.75 D from target and the patient is complaining.
- Visual acuity uncorrected of 20/40 or worse in the distance eye—in other words, the patient is no longer 20/happy.
- Astigmatism causing symptoms and greater than 0.75′ D. Symptoms are usually described as shadows or double-images.

Some general retreatment statistics from Hunkeler Eye Centers:

- Of patients with more than 1 D of cylinder, 90% need enhancement.
- Of patients with 1 D of cylinder, 40% need enhancement.
- Of patients with less than 1 D of cylinder, 10% need enhancement.

A study by Stulting et al.[2] including 1,062 LASIK procedures showed that only 5.3% of the eyes had complications. Of all their retreated eyes, only 3.9% had complications. Daniel Durrie, MD, a refractive surgeon at Hunkeler Eye Centers, believes that retreatment after LASIK may be safer than the original procedure. He also believes advances in technology will make this procedure safer. Hunkeler-NovaMed Centers' experience with the Hansatome microkeratome (Bausch & Lomb, Rochester, NY) has proven to significantly reduce serious LASIK flap complications. (D. Durrie, *personal communication*, 1999). After 8,344 procedures performed by eight different surgeons using the Hansatome, they have not experienced any flap-related complications or epithelial ingrowth. This also includes the 5.7% who were retreated. Increased safety features of this microkeratome include automatic stop if suction is lost, easier assembly, and a permanent depth plate setting.

There are symptoms that the patient experiences postoperatively that should not be interpreted as complications. These symptoms include dryness, fluctuating vision, and night-time glare and halos. Many refractive surgery patients have dry eye symptoms up to 6 months. This may be secondary to nerve regeneration or disruption of the tear film. Fluctuating vision and nighttime glare and halos are common symptoms for approximately 1 month after the procedure. These are only temporary symptoms, and the clinician would be wise to explain these occurrences before surgery.

References

1. Smith RJ, Maloney RK. Diffuse lamellar keratitis. A new syndrome in lamellar refractive surgery. Ophthalmology 1998;105:1721–1726.
2. Stulting RD, Carr JD, Thompson KP, et al. Ophthalmology 1999;106:13–19.
3. Wilson SE. LASIK: management of common complications. Cornea 1998;17: 459–467.
4. Farah SG, Azar DT, Gurdal C, Wong J. Laser in situ keratomileusis: literature review of a developing technique. J Cataract Refract Surg 1998;24:989–1006.
5. Davidorf JM, Zaldivar R, Oscherow S. Results and complications of laser in situ keratomileusis by experienced surgeons. J Refract Surg 1998;14:114–122.

CHAPTER 9

Outcomes

Milton M. Hom

Numerous factors affect the outcomes of LASIK. Variables such as methods of preoperative refraction, room temperature and humidity, room air quality and flow, surgical technique and time, and postoperative medications can influence the outcomes.[1] For other procedures, such as intraocular lens (IOL) implants, the outcomes are much more precise than refractive surgery. For example, the refractive effect of a standard cataract procedure with an uncomplicated placement of the IOL can be identical for two different surgeons; however, the same cannot be said for LASIK.[2]

Pearl:
For IOL placement, the refractive effect can be identical for two surgeons. The same cannot be said for LASIK.

During the preoperative workup, the true refractive error must be determined. The co-managing practitioner needs to make certain the proper vertex distance is taken into account.[2] This can be especially significant, because many LASIK patients have high refractive errors. The vertex distance can be rechecked with a trial frame measurement (see Chapter 4, Preprocedure Selection and Workup). Cycloplegic refraction must also be considered to eliminate overminusing. The laser ablates the target refraction entered into the computer. If the refractive data are incorrect, a residual refractive error results. The difference between the true refraction and the refraction entered into the computer is usually what makes up the residual refractive error.[2]

Algorithm

The laser is computer-controlled. The part of the software that determines the ablation pattern is called the *algorithm*. Each laser system has a different algorithm, depending on the desired beam delivery and beam fluence. Beam delivery varies with the ablation zone diameter. Beam fluence is the energy per pulse that is distributed over a defined area.[2]

Beam delivery is also influenced by the *Munnerlyn formula*. The Munnerlyn formula relates the depth of correction to the amount of correction and ablation zone:

$$\text{depth of ablation} = \frac{\text{diopters of correction} \times \text{ablation diameter}^2}{3}$$

A good rule of thumb is for a 6-mm ablation zone, 12 µm in depth are needed for every diopter of correction.[1] The programming for the ablation varies for each type of laser system. Pretreatment protocols and the type and number of ablation zones influence ablation depth. Pretreatments are largely used to avoid central island formation. However, pretreatment greatly increases the ablation depth. For low corrections (1–2 D), the VISX Staar and Chiron Technolas Keracor 116 require a depth of 17–20 µm per D. When a multipass, multizone ablation is used, the ablation depth needed per diopter is significantly reduced.[1] An example is the VISX Staar international card, a multipass, multizoned ablation that reduces the depth needed to 10 µm per D.[1]

The predictive formulas for LASIK have two components: the nomogram and the adjustment factors.[1] The ablation nomogram controls the distribution of refraction correction into each of the ablation zones. The adjustment factors further refine the customization process. The nomogram and adjustment factors should be tailored for each surgeon.[1] By tracking outcomes, the surgeon determines his or her own nomogram to program the laser. Because of the variability of surgical technique and laser centers, nomograms are usually not exactly alike. To get an identical outcome between two surgeons, two different nomograms are needed. Establishing a proper nomogram increases the predictability of LASIK.

Nomogram

The nomogram takes several considerations into account. Amounts of preoperative refractive error, age, and healing patterns are prominent factors. There are greater amounts of regression for higher amounts of myopia.[1] With respect to age, patients younger than 25 years often demonstrate significant regression. Patients older than age 50 years may not show any regression at all. Age is usually taken into account as an adjustment factor. The healing pattern can also differ between two eyes for the same patient. There are cases in which one eye has 1–2 D of regression, and the companion eye has no regression. The bilateral procedures were performed one after the other, using the same surgical technique and identical nomograms and adjustment factors. Sometimes, different healing patterns are difficult to predict.[1]

Pearl:
The unpredictable pattern of healing represents the limitation of refractive surgery.[1]

Adjustment Factors

Altitude of the refractive center and patient age are the two most commonly considered adjustment factors.[1] Altitude has an effect on the station pressure or barometric readings of the refractive center. The excimer laser emits controlled pulses of ultraviolet light. The ultraviolet light is a product of an inert gas and a halide. The *Ideal Gas Law* solved for density is $D = P/(T \times R)$, where D represents density; P represents station pressure; T represents temperature (K); and R represents the gas constant. Temperature and air density (related to humidity) are usually well controlled in the laser room. This leaves station pressure or barometric reading as the remaining variable.[1]

Patient age is another adjustment factor. A slight overcorrection of 0.5 D is preferable for patients younger than 25 years. A slight amount of hyperopic drift (undercorrection) is expected. Patients older than 50 years are undercorrected by 0.50 D.[1] A comparison of different nomograms is shown in Table 9.1. The table shows that each surgeon adjusts the algorithm by a certain percentage based on his or her own situation.

Surgical technique has a great influence on the ablation. As discussed earlier (see Chapter 6, Description of Primary Procedure and Retreatment), there are different techniques for wetting and drying the cornea, stromal bed, and flap. The frequency, timing, amount of wiping during ablation, and use of forced air are just a few of the influencing factors. The hydration state of the stroma also determines how much tissue is removed for the same number of pulses. More tissue is removed for a drier bed, and less tissue is removed for a wetter bed.[2]

Pearl:
The drier the bed, the more tissue is removed.[2]

As stated in Chapter 6, LASIK has been described as 90% keratectomy and 10% laser; however, patients strongly desire 100% keratectomy success followed by 100% laser ablation success. An optimized nomogram brings the laser portion of the surgery closer to the desired outcome.[2]

Pearl:
The three important elements in establishing a nomogram are the laser, the laser room environment, and the surgical technique.[2]

TABLE 9.1
Nomogram Comparison

Surgeon	Location	Enhancement Rate (%)	Preoperative MR Rate (D)	Altitude (Ft)	Temperature Range (°F)	Humidity Range (%)	Drying	Age Adjustment	Sphere Adjustment (%)	Cylinder Adjustment (%)
1	Tulsa, OK	21	1–16	711	60–65	30–40	—	—	10	—
2	Oklahoma City, OK	10	1–17	1,208	65–70	40–60	—	—	20	—
3	Garden City, NY	15	1–16	0	65–76	30–60	Subjective	Yes	Sliding: 14–18	10
4	Seattle, WA	5	1–15	0	60–65	30–40	—	—	7.7	—
5	Brea, CA	8	0.75–13.75	650	60–70	45–50	Periodic	—	8	—
6	Indianapolis, IN	8	1–15	770	60–65	35–40	Periodic	Yes	20	—
7	Denver, CO	25	1–20	5,280	60–65	35–45	—	—	30	—
8	Rockville, MD	15	0.75–16.00	0	60–65	35–45	—	Yes	Sliding: 15–20	—
9	Fairfax, VA	15	0.75–16.00	0	60–65	35–40	—	Yes	Sliding: 15–20	—
10	New York, NY	10	0.5–22.0	0	60–68	30–35	—	Yes	Sliding: 10–20	—

11	Charlotte, NC	15	1–16	765	60–70	35–40	—	—	15	—
12	Rockville, MD	15	1–16	0	60–65	35–40	—	Yes	15	10
13	Fairfax, VA	7	1–16	0	60–65	35–40	—	Yes	15	10
14	Greenville, SC	10	1–16	950	60–70	35–50	Subjective	—	10	—
15	Johnson City, TN	10	1–16	1,700	60–70	30–45	Subjective	—	20	—

Source: Data from LE Probst, J Woolfson, M Kritzinger. Predictive Formulas for LASIK. In: JJ Machat, SG Slade, LE Probst (eds), The Art of LASIK (2nd ed). Thorofare, NJ: Slack, 1999;59.

Visual Outcomes

There have been many studies on the effectiveness of LASIK. One study shows that 46.4% of the eyes at 6 months had uncorrected visual acuity of 20/40 or better.[2] More recent studies show improvement in outcomes to 93.6% within 0.43 D for myopia and within 0.33 D for astigmatism.[3]

The Emory Vision Correction Center, in Atlanta, found that 92% of eyes achieved 20/40 or better, and that 42.1% saw 20/20 or better.[4] In its Nidek study, which included toric ablations, 85% achieved 20/40 or better, and 44.9% achieved 20/20 or better.[4] The CRS study found that 81% had 20/40 or better with the Summit Apex and 85% with the VISX Staar.[5] At the London Laser Center, 91% of eyes achieved 20/20 or better, and 50% of the eyes achieved 20/20 or better.[6]

A literature review of LASIK studies revealed that the average refractive error treated was –8.71 D, yielding a mean postoperative refraction of +0.93D. An average of 82.5% of eyes were within ± 1 D of emmetropia. Postoperative best corrected visual acuity averaged 83.2% for 20/40 or better and 48% for 20/20 or better. Postoperative uncorrected visual acuity averaged 83.2% for 20/40 or better and 56.6% for 20/20 or better. Only 0.9% of the eyes lost two or more lines of vision (Table 9.2).[7] When reviewing the literature on visual outcomes, recent abstracts show significant improvements over those described in older literature. The recent abstracts strongly suggest that there is continual improvement in the procedure.[7]

Pearl:
Visual outcomes show significant strides when recent abstracts are compared with published papers. This indicates a rapidly improving technique.[7]

Hyperopia

For hyperopia, the procedure is much newer. Although the outcomes do not yet have the benefit of experience when compared to myopic LASIK, the results are excellent.[8] Early studies divide the results according to preoperative amount. In one study, for 2 D or less of hyperopia, 94.1% of the cases achieved 20/40 or better uncorrected visual acuity. Between 2 and 3 D, 100% had uncorrected visual acuity of 20/40 or better. For higher than 3 D, 87.8% had uncorrected visual acuity 20/40 or better.[9] In other studies, uncorrected visual acuity of 20/40 or better was obtained by 90–95% of the eyes.[10,11] Arbelaz showed hyperopic LASIK to be effective for up to 4 D, whereas others target hyperopia upwards to 5–6 D.[8,11,12]

The hyperopic ablation profile requires a steepened periphery. One difficulty lies in the small optic zone, resulting in halos and glare (see Chapter 6, Description of Primary Procedure and Retreatment). As the procedure

TABLE 9.2
Outcomes of LASIK

First Author	Number of Eyes	Within 1 D	Postoperative Best Corrected Visual Acuity >20/40 (%)	Postoperative Best Corrected Visual Acuity >20/20(%)	Postoperative Uncorrected Visual Acuity >20/40 (%)	Postoperative Uncorrected Vision >20/20 (%)	Loss of Two or More Lines (%)
Burrato[13]	30	80	80	6	0	0	—
Burrato[14]	150	85.3	15.3	0.66	0	0	8
Burrato[15]	30	57	80	6.7	10	0	3.3
Pallikaris[16]	10	66.6	—	—	—	—	—
Brint[17]	47	—	—	—	65.9	34.1	21.3
Bas[18]	97	46.5	77	—	49.9	—	13
Fiander[19]	124	70	—	—	81	50	—
Kremer[20]	5	—	—	—	—	—	20
Slade[21]	57	47.8	—	—	66	—	6.4
Kremer[22]	31	74.2	—	—	81	—	0
Salah[23]	59	73	—	—	76	44	10
Guell[24]	21	85	71.4	14.3	71.4	0	0
	22	41	50	4.5	45	0	—
Helmy[25]	40	85.7	100	60	75	17.5	—
Mainho[26]	34	67.6	—	—	—	—	8.82
Salah[27]	88	72	88	44.6	71	36	3.6
Kim[28]	18	47	—	—	—	—	5.5
Gimbel[29]	5	—	100	—	100	—	0
	32	—	100	—	50	—	15

Continued

TABLE 9.2 (continued)

First Author	Number of Eyes	Within 1 D	Postoperative Best Corrected Visual Acuity >20/40 (%)	Postoperative Best Corrected Visual Acuity >20/20(%)	Postoperative Uncorrected Visual Acuity >20/40 (%)	Postoperative Uncorrected Vision >20/20 (%)	Loss of Two or More Lines (%)
	11	—	63	—	36	—	27
	5	—	20	—	0	—	40
Knorz[30]	51	47	96	—	29.2	7.8	12
Arenas[31]	4	—	50	0	0	0	—
Condon[32]	51	—	—	—	—	—	—
Pallikaris[33]	21	—	—	—	—	—	—
	18	—	—	—	—	—	—
Perez-Santonja[34]	143	60	—	—	46.4	—	1.4
Mean		67	64	21	49.2	22	8
ISRS 1996 abstracts	3,995	84 (368 cases)	92 (250 cases)	—	89 (423 cases)	36 (32 cases)	2 (4 cases)
ACSRS 1997 abstracts	5,412	90.9 (502 cases)	90.96 (1,356 cases)	48 (1,299 cases)	83.3 (555 cases)	90 (98 cases)	0.9 (1,011 cases)
ARVO 1997 abstracts	1,990	67.4 (311 cases)	—	—	71 (198 cases)	50.2 (311 cases)	—
Mean		82.5	91.2	48	83.2	56.6	0.9

(—) indicates the information is unclear, not mentioned, or not quantified.
ARVO = Association for Research in Vision and Ophthalmology; ASCRS = American Society of Cataract and Refractive Surgery; ISRS = International Society for Refractive Surgery.
Source: Data from SG Farah, DT Azar, C Gurdal, J Wong. Laser in situ keratomileusis: literature review of a developing technique. J Cataract Refract Surg 1998;24:994–995.

improves, the refractive envelope of hyperopic LASIK will widen and effectiveness should increase.

References

1. Probst LE, Woolfson J, Kritzinger M. Predictive Formulas for LASIK. In JJ Machat, SG Slade, LE Probst (eds), The Art of LASIK (2nd ed). Thorofare, NJ: Slack, 1999;55–63.
2. Doane JF. Personalized LASIK Nomogram Development. In JJ Machat, SG Slade, LE Probst (eds), The Art of LASIK (2nd ed). Thorofare, NJ: Slack, 1999; 65–78.
3. El Danasoruy MA, Waring GO, El-Maghraby A, et al. Excimer laser in situ keratomileusis to correct compound myopic astigmatism. J Refract Surg 1997;13:511–520.
4. Carr JD, Thompson KP, Stulting RD, Waring GO. LASIK: Emory Vision Correction Center. In JJ Machat, SG Slade, LE Probst (eds), The Art of LASIK (2nd ed). Thorofare, NJ: Slack, 1999;281–292.
5. Kezirian GM, Casebeer JC. The CRS LASIK Study. In JJ Machat, SG Slade, LE Probst (eds), The Art of LASIK (2nd ed). Thorofare, NJ: Slack, 1999;293–302.
6. Probst LE, Hakim OJ, Nichols BD, Baird M. LASIK Results from TLC, The London Laser Center. In JJ Machat, SG Slade, LE Probst (eds), The Art of LASIK (2nd ed). Thorofare, NJ: Slack, 1999;303–308.
7. Farah SG, Azar DT, Gurdal C, Wong J. Laser in situ keratomileusis: literature review of a developing technique. J Cataract Refract Surg 1998;24:989–1006.
8. Arbelaez MC. Hyperopic LASIK with the Chiron Technolas Excimer Laser. In JJ Machat, SG Slade, LE Probst (eds), The Art of LASIK (2nd ed). Thorofare, NJ: Slack, 1999;311–315.
9. Argento CJ, Cosentino MJ. Laser in situ keratomileusis for hyperopia. J Cataract Refract Surg 1998;24:1050–1058.
10. Buzard KA, Fundingsland BR. Excimer laser in situ keratomileusis for hyperopia. J Cataract Refract Surg 1999;25:197–204.
11. Ditzen K, Huschka H, Pieger S. Laser in situ keratomileusis for hyperopia. J Cataract Refract Surg 1998;24:42–47.
12. Lawless MA, Sutton GI. Hyperopic LASIK with the Summit Apex Plus Laser. In JJ Machat, SG Slade, LE Probst (eds), The Art of LASIK (2nd ed). Thorofare, NJ: Slack, 1999;317–321.
13. Burrato L, Ferrari M, Rama P. Excimer laser intrastromal keratomileusis. Am J Ophthalmol 1992;113:291–295.
14. Burrato L, Ferrari M, Genisi C. Keratomileusis for myopia with the excimer laser (Burrato technique): short term results. Refract Corneal Surg 1993;9: S130–S133.
15. Burrato L, Ferrari M, Genisi C. Myopic keratomileusis with the excimer laser: one year follow-up. Refract Corneal Surg 1993;9:12–19.

16. Pallikaris IG, Signos DS. Excimer laser in situ keratomileusis and photorefractive keratectomy for correction of high myopia. J Refract Corneal Surg 1994;10:498–510.
17. Brint SF, Ostrick DM, Fisher C, et al. Six-month results of the multicenter phase 1 study of the excimer laser myopic keratomileusis. J Cataract Refract Surg 1994;20:610–615.
18. Bas AM, Onnis R. Excimer laser in situ keratomileusis for myopia. J Refract Surg 1995;11:S229–S233.
19. Fiander DC, Trayfour F. Excimer laser in situ keratomileusis in 124 myopic eyes. J Refract Surg 1995;11:S234–S238.
20. Kremer I, Blumenthal M. Myopic keratomileusis in situ combined with VISX 20/20 photorefractive keratectomy. J Cataract Refract Surg 1995;21:508–511.
21. Slade SG, Brint SF, Updegraff SA. Excimer Laser Myopic Keratomileusis: United States Experience. In JJ Salz (ed), Corneal Laser Surgery. St. Louis: Mosby, 1995;195–196.
22. Kremer FB, Dufek M. Excimer laser in situ keratomileusis. J Refract Surg 1995;11:S244–S247.
23. Salah T, Waring GO III, El-Maghraby A. Excimer Laser Keratomileusis in the Corneal Bed Under a Hinged Flap: Results in Saudi Arabia at the El-Maghraby Eye Hospital. In JJ Salz (ed), Corneal Laser Surgery. St. Louis: Mosby, 1995;187–195.
24. Guell JL, Muller A. Laser in situ keratomileusis (LASIK) for myopia from –7 to –18 diopters. J Refract Surg 1996;12:222–228.
25. Helmy SA, Salah A, Badawy T, Sidky AN. Photorefractive keratectomy and laser in situ keratomileusis for myopia between 6.00 and 10.00 diopters. J Refract Surg 1996;12:417–421.
26. Marinho A, Pinto MC, Pinto R, et al. LASIK for high myopia: one year experience. Ophthalmic Surg Lasers 1996;27:S517–S520.
27. Salah T, Waring GO III, El-Maghraby A, et al. Excimer laser keratomileusis in the corneal bed under a hinged flap for myopia of 2 to 20 diopters. Am J Ophthalmol 1996;121:143–155.
28. Kim H-M, Juung HR. Laser assisted in situ keratomileusis for high myopia. Ophthalmic Surg Lasers 1996;27:S508–S511.
29. Gimbel HV, Basti S, Kaye GB, Ferenspwicz M. Experience during the learning curve of laser in situ keratomileusis. J Cataract Refract Surg 1996;22:542–550.
30. Knorz MC, Liermann A, Seiberth V, et al. Laser in situ keratomileusis to correct myopia of –6.00 to –29.00 diopters. J Refract Surg 1996;12:575–584.
31. Arenas E, Maglione A. Laser in situ keratomileusis for astigmatism and myopia after penetrating keratoplasty. J Refract Surg 1997;13:27–32.
32. Condon PI, Mulhern M, Fulcher T, et al. Laser intrastromal keratomileusis for high myopia and myopic astigmatism. Br J Ophthalmol 1997;81:199–206.
33. Pallikaris IG, Siganos DS. Laser in situ keratomileusis to treat myopia: early experience. J Cataract Refract Surg 1997;23:39–49.
34. Perez-Santonja JJ, Bellot J, Claramonte P, et al. Laser in situ keratomileusis to correct high myopia. J Cataract Refract Surg 1997;23:372–385.

CHAPTER 10

Corneal Topography and Contact Lenses After LASIK

Loretta B. Szczotka

With LASIK becoming the preferred refractive procedure around the world, increasing numbers of primary eye care and contact lens practitioners are confronted with postoperative LASIK patients. The increasing numbers of LASIK procedures will eventually require contact lens considerations in a subgroup of these patients, mandating new approaches to traditional contact lens fittings. Because the corneal shape has been significantly altered from the contour for which the contact lenses were originally designed, new lens designs and fitting techniques are often required for optimal contact lens performance. Patients with a satisfactory visual result may request contact lens correction for further visual enhancement, cosmetic use, or eventual presbyopic demands. Patients with postoperative complications resulting in suboptimal visual results can present early or late in the postoperative phase for visual improvement with contact lenses.

Most suboptimal visual outcomes include under- and overcorrections and do not involve a loss of best corrected spectacle acuity. Patients seeking refractive surgery for the purpose of discontinuing spectacle wear often pursue contact lenses in cases in which significant ametropia remains. The greatest percentage of patients in my practice presenting for contact lens correction after refractive surgery are those who had radial keratotomy (RK) when it was popular in the early 1980s. Many of these patients, most of whom are now presbyopic, are symptomatic from overcorrections and hyperopic drifts since their original procedure. Ten years after the Prospective Evaluation of Radial Keratotomy Study, 58% of the study patients thought some type of optical correction was required; 23% of patients had overcorrections or induced hyperopia greater than 1 D, and 17% had undercorrections or residual myopia greater than 1 D.[1] Since the shift to a primary or augmented use of the excimer laser in most refractive techniques, fewer photorefractive keratotomy (PRK) and LASIK patients proceed to contact lens fitting compared to RK because of greater predictability and accu-

Chapter modified from LB Szczotka, M Aronsky. Contact lenses after LASIK. J Am Optom Assoc 1998;69:775–784.

racy. However, complications such as over- and undercorrections still exist. One year after LASIK, in a study of patients with moderate myopic astigmatism, the authors reported a 5.4% overcorrection rate between +0.75 and +1.25 D, and a 15% undercorrection rate between –1.00 and –2.13 D.[2] In high myopia, one study reported overcorrections greater than +1.00 D in 17.3% of eyes and undercorrections greater than –1.5 D in 15.2% of eyes 6 months after LASIK surgery.[3]

Excimer laser procedures have also decreased visual complication rates compared to incisional procedures. Postoperative RK patients experienced complications such as visual fluctuations secondary to changes in stromal hydration; glare induced by incisions within the visual axis; and irregular astigmatism from eccentric optical zones, uneven healing, unintentional incisions crossing the entrance pupil, micro- or macroperforations, or intersecting radial and tangential incisions.[4,5] Although less common after LASIK, suboptimal visual performance may also be associated with irregular astigmatism, glare, and halos. Irregular astigmatism after LASIK has been reported with incidences from 1.1% to 11% and is either a result of a decentered ablation, a decentered flap, persistent central islands, cap misalignment or loss, corneal perforation, epithelial ingrowth, corneal melting, interface inflammation, or, rarely, interface haze.[3,6,7] Glare (starbursts) has been reported to occur as frequently as 31.5% after LASIK for high myopia and is most often caused by corneal haze.[2,3] (The term *haze* in LASIK describes the degree of decreased clarity of the interface rather than subepithelial haze reported after PRK.[8]) Halos have been reported to occur in up to 29% of patients after LASIK for high myopia and are associated with small ablation diameters.[3] Irregular astigmatism can be easily managed with rigid gas-permeable (RGP) contact lenses, although glare and halos may still persist after RGP lens wear.

Although LASIK's primary purpose is to eliminate the dependence on spectacle or contact lens wear, some patients are encouraged to seek contact lens alternatives because they easily manage unanticipated over- or undercorrections or irregular astigmatism. Fitting contact lenses to the LASIK patient with an unanticipated visual result can be challenging because of the physical attributes of the cornea as well as the psychological attributes of the patient. The selection of contact lenses depends on the time after surgery, mode of lens wear, degree of corneal irregularity, and best corrected spectacle acuity.

Contact Lens Management

PREFITTING ANALYSIS

Because most patients proceeding to elective LASIK surgery have been pre-screened for concurrent external ocular diseases, they should have no specific contraindications to contact lens wear. After PRK, knowledge of the early healing response is important in fitting contact lenses because it gives the contact lens fitter a good indication of the integrity of the patient's epithelium and stroma. For example, classification into one of the three healing responses identified after PRK is helpful because it may encourage or contraindicate future contact lens wear, or it may dictate the selection of postoperative lens alternatives. After LASIK, the healing response is not as important as in PRK. In LASIK, no stromal healing types have been identified, although there may be a slight tendency of a myopic drift (<1 D) in some highly myopic patients without haze formation (i.e., regression without haze). Refractions are relatively stable 4–12 weeks after LASIK, and a soft contact lens can be fit as early as the refraction is stable for those patients who are not candidates for surgical enhancements or refuse further procedures to correct the residual ametropia.[3,8] In high myopia (> –16.00 D), refractions may not be stable until 6 months or more, indicating corneal flap healing is not complete, and all contact lens fitting should be postponed until a consistent refraction is achieved.[3,8]

Although there is no way to measure the stability of a corneal flap before RGP fitting (except stability in refraction and topography), rigid lenses have been safely fit 8–12 weeks after surgery. Most surgeons agree that the integrity of the flap after 3 months is sufficient to withstand the minor trauma and movement of an RGP lens. By 3 months, refractions and corneal thickness changes stabilize and corneal sensitivity returns to its preoperative values.[3,8,9]

Soft Lenses

Patients often request hydrophilic contact lenses to correct residual refractive error, especially in cases of presurgical RGP intolerance. After RK, long-term wear of soft lenses should be avoided because their chronic use has been reported to account for neovascularization along the incision lines. After LASIK or PRK, the use of soft lenses to correct residual ametropias is more accepted. Because there are no incisions in the postoperative PRK eye and only superficial incisions paracentrally after LASIK, complication rates of corneal neovascularization from soft lens–induced hypoxia are similar to nonsurgical eyes.

After PRK, bandage hydrogel contact lenses are widely prescribed in the immediate postoperative phase to protect the loosely adhered, healing epithelium. Ciba Vision Ophthalmics (Duluth, GA) has developed the Pro-Tek Lens (vifilcon A, 55% water) for this purpose, an ionic hydrogel intentionally designed as a postoperative PRK bandage. It incorporates an ultrathin center and base curves of 8.9 or 9.2 mm to better conform to the oblate PRK contour. Standard, extended-wear disposable lenses have also been used with good results, although they have not been specifically approved by the U.S. Food and Drug Administration for therapeutic purposes.[10,11] After LASIK, most of the epithelium remains intact; therefore, bandage lenses are not widely prescribed postoperatively. Some surgeons, however, still use bandage lenses on the first postoperative day to speed flap margin re-epithelialization and to protect against potential trauma from the eyelid.[12] Generally, bandage lenses are not recommended after LASIK, and their use has been associated with increased epithelial distortion, corneal edema, and delayed visual rehabilitation.[12] Their use should be reserved for treatment of an unanticipated epithelial defect or to avoid corneal damage from eyelid abnormalities during the early postoperative period. Additionally, after LASIK enhancements, some surgeons now use bandage soft lenses in the early postoperative phase to prevent epithelial ingrowth through the disrupted epithelial flap edge.

After LASIK, almost all corneas result in oblate contours, characterized by flatter central corneal curvatures and steeper peripheries (Figure 10.1). Currently, only one soft lens is designed and approved by the U.S. Food and Drug Administration for the correction of ametropias after refractive surgeries that result in oblate corneal shapes. The Harrison Post Refractive Lens (Paragon Vision Sciences, Mesa, AZ) is indicated for patients whose corneal topography has been altered after RK, PRK, LASIK, and other refractive procedures that produce flattened central corneal contours with steeper peripheries. The lens functions like a reverse geometry design that incorporates a central optical portion that is flatter than the midperiphery. Although a reverse geometry lens design is critical for suc-

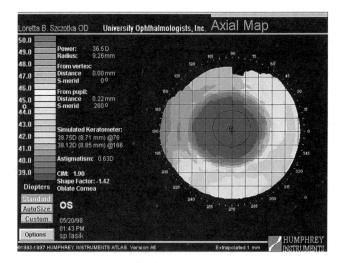

FIGURE 10.1. Oblate LASIK corneal shape. (Courtesy of LB Szczotka, M Aronsky. Contact lenses after LASIK. J Am Optom Assoc 1998;69:775–784.)

cess when fitting RGP lenses to some oblate corneas, the use of such a design in soft lenses may not be as important. Most soft lenses drape over the underlying corneal contour, especially ultrathin disposable lenses; therefore, novel back-surface designs are not a significant factor in the selection of a spherical soft lenses after LASIK. Many standard disposables have been fit with success.

For the patient with residual regular astigmatism, soft toric lenses are often considered, especially if the patient was previously RGP intolerant and pursued refractive surgery to eliminate RGP wear. Mixed astigmatism (hyperopia and minus cylinder astigmatism) is a common postoperative refractive error after LASIK and becomes symptomatic as the patient enters presbyopia. If a patient desires contact lenses instead of spectacles for visual enhancement, soft toric lenses are a good option; however, they can be more difficult to fit on postoperative corneas compared to preoperative corneas because of unexpected lens back-surface-to-cornea fitting relationships. Empirical fitting of soft torics is not recommended because of occasional atypical rotational stability and unpredictable lens rotation on oblate corneal shapes. Diagnostic lens fitting is highly encouraged to assess lens stability and rotation so that the appropriate axis compensation can be performed if needed.

RIGID GAS-PERMEABLE LENSES

The lens of choice after LASIK is an RGP lens because of material rigidity, high oxygen transmissibility, removal of corneal by-products and tear debris through efficient tear exchange, and neutralization of corneal irregularity through the formation of a posterior lens tear pool. The perceived difficulty in fitting RGP lenses after LASIK is associated with the postoperative oblate corneal shape, which is one of the most difficult corneal contours to fit with standard RGP designs and fitting techniques. Although standard RGP designs are often used successfully, new fitting guidelines are required because the traditional RGP fitting nomograms, originally designed for prolate corneal contours (steeper in the center and flatter in the periphery), are not appropriate for lens base curve or optical zone selection after LASIK. Additionally, lens power calculations may be altered from traditional or empirical lens fitting nomograms because of an unpredictable tear clearance and lacrimal lens formation above the ablation zone. Although corneal topography systems are beneficial and recommended when fitting RGP lenses, their associated contact lens modules have not been proved on postsurgical eyes. Often their lens power and base curve recommendations are inaccurate because of inappropriate tear layer simulations; therefore, trial lens fitting is mandatory, especially to determine lens power, base curve, and optical zone diameters.

Pearl:
The lens of choice after LASIK is an RGP lens due to its material rigidity.

As in standard RGP fitting, the most comfortable RGP fit occurs when the lens rests in a slightly superior position and receives support from the upper lid or is perfectly centered over the surgical optical zone. Lens movement will vary with the fitting approach. A lid attachment fit may move <1 mm with each blink, whereas an interpalpebral-centered fit may move significantly more depending on the lens diameter. The contact lens vaults the flatter corneal surgical zone centrally, resulting in fluorescein pooling and a plus-powered lacrimal lens (Figure 10.2). This plus-powered tear layer must be compensated for by adding additional minus power in the RGP lens, resulting in a lens power that approaches the patient's preoperative sphere power. The lens will rest paracentrally on the highest point of elevation, which is the bend in the corneal contour, surrounding the flattened ablation zone. This area is referred to as the *inflection zone* or *point*. There should be minimal fluorescein accumulation over the inflection zones, with 1- to 2-mm wide bands of midperipheral bearing. Peripheral edge lift should be sufficient to prevent peripheral adherence and seal off but not too high to promote a break in the tear meniscus. A standard 0.12-mm axial edge lift, common to standard RGP fitting techniques, should be sufficient.

Because the peripheral cornea is essentially unchanged after LASIK (as well as PRK), RGP lens fitting is simple compared to postoperative RK lens fitting, in which corneal incisions induce direct shape changes in the periphery. After RK, asymmetric steepening surrounding the surgical optical zone may affect lens centration, which is not usually encountered after LASIK. There is often improved RGP centration after LASIK compared to a patient's preoperative RGP lens performance because of increased negative pressure created by the steep central tear layer.[13]

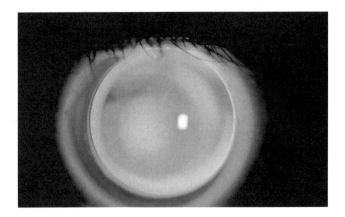

FIGURE 10.2. Acceptable rigid gas–permeable fit and fluorescein pattern after LASIK.

Pearl:
RGP centration is often improved after LASIK because of the increased negative pressure created by the steep central tear layer.

CORNEAL CURVATURE ASSESSMENT AND RIGID GAS-PERMEABLE LENS BASE CURVE SELECTION

After LASIK, initial RGP base curve selection for standard lens designs varies depending on the method of corneal curvature assessment: preoperative keratometry, postoperative keratometry, or postoperative corneal topography.

Some fitters advocate the use of standard RGP designs after excimer laser procedures instead of reverse geometry lenses designed for oblate corneal shapes. In one series of postoperative PRK patients, all eyes studied were successfully fit postoperatively with standard aspheric designs.[13] Final RGP base curves were fitted on average 0.065 mm flatter than the preoperative RGP lens, and several lenses were fit with the same RGP base curve as was worn preoperatively. Preoperative keratometry, or K readings from the preoperative eye, can be a reasonable predictor of initial diagnostic lens base curves after PRK or LASIK. If using presurgical keratometry, the initial trial base curve selected should be 0.5–1.0 D flatter than flat K to account for the surgically induced flattened central cornea.[14] The base curve can be steepened if the fit is too flat with excessive peripheral liftoff, or flattened if the lens fits too steep with excessive peripheral impingement and central pooling (Figure 10.3).

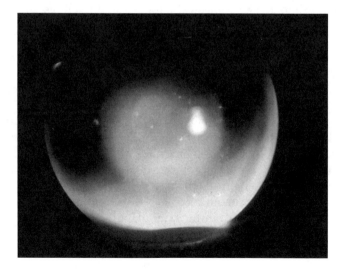

FIGURE 10.3. Unacceptable steep rigid gas-permeable fit and fluorescein pattern after LASIK.

Central postoperative K readings may mislead the selection of an initial trial lens base curve due to the surgically flattened central corneal values and are not recommended as the primary measurement for base curve selection; however, postoperative keratometry readings are often the only measurements available. One study reported that lens fitting based on flat postoperative keratometry readings was acceptable after refractive surgery such as RK, although most of the final base curves were ultimately steeper than the postoperative flat K when the fitting was completed.[15] In our experience, due to the disproportionate amount of central corneal flattening and relative peripheral steepening after RK, PRK, or LASIK compared to a preoperative eye, a contact lens fit near the average or flat central postoperative K will be unacceptably flat and unstable because of little or no midperipheral bearing. The initial lens chosen should be, at minimum, 1.0–1.5 D steeper than the flat K postoperatively. This lens fit is then refined to achieve the goal of midperipheral corneal alignment and central pooling.

A better postoperative keratometry fitting technique uses revised peripheral keratometry readings.[16] This technique provides an estimation of the midperipheral curvature approximately 3 mm from the center of the cornea. Four fixation dots are placed symmetrically 4 mm from the horizontal and vertical edges of the keratometer viewing port, and as the patient changes fixation onto each target dot, the nasal, temporal, superior, and inferior midperipheral readings are recorded. Although this technique is simple to perform, the exact corneal location of the points being measured is still uncertain. When fitting RGP lenses, some fitters suggest selecting the initial base curve equal to the temporal reading, which should provide a lens with midperipheral corneal alignment and central tear pooling, although others have averaged the four lateral readings with successful results.[16,17]

Corneal topography is the most sophisticated method of assessing corneal curvatures after refractive surgery and is possibly the most appropriate method for contact lens fitting. The most important data retrievable from topography systems for RGP contact lens fitting include a preliminary shape classification, the optical zone size, simulated central keratometry, midperipheral corneal curvature, and the dioptric curvature change across the surgical transition zone.

Corneal topography software programs allow a variety of map displays that vary in their application of proprietary algorithms to the raw data. The two most informative shape displays used for contact lens fitting after refractive surgery are the instantaneous radius of curvature maps (i.e., tangential, local, or true maps) and the axial distance maps (i.e., sagittal, color, or default maps). The axial distance maps do not actually represent true corneal curvatures. The axial algorithms produce spherically biased reference distances that became the standard displays in most early corneal topography systems. The instantaneous radius of curvature maps produces *true* curvatures based on a standard definition of the local curvature at a given point along a curve. Both instantaneous and axial representations offer qualitatively similar views of corneal shape, but instantaneous maps provide smaller and more centrally located patterns than axial maps and include extreme curvature values. Axial maps produce a running average of the analyzed data for a given peripheral location and therefore exclude extreme curvature values, offering a more global representation of corneal shape.

Differences between the two representations of curvature become significant for corneal points away from the reference (optical) axis or specifically in the mid to far corneal periphery. These differences become clinically relevant after LASIK because the shape changes produced in the midperiphery, such as over the bend or transition of the ablation zone, begin to differ significantly between the two representations, which can directly affect the selection of RGP contact lens parameters. Color Plate 7 shows a postoperative LASIK eye imaged by both the instantaneous and axial reconstruction algorithms. Note that the cursor positioned over the same location within the transition zone on each map reads values that differ by more than 7 D. Roberts documented the abrupt curvature changes and oblate patterns after RK apparent on corneal topography maps and the differences between midperipheral corneal curvatures when comparing axial and instantaneous reconstruction algorithms.[18] Similar patterns are found on topography maps after LASIK, in which instantaneous radius of curvature maps display a very defined, steep transitional ring surrounding the central flat zone, but on axial maps only a central flat zone may be noted due to the averaging nature of the axial algorithm (Color Plate 8).

If standard spherical RGP lenses are fit postoperatively, then the topographic averaged axial curvatures, based on spherically biased algorithms, should provide the most relevant data for posterior RGP curvature selection. McDonnell and colleagues selected data points from computerized corneal topography maps as an aid in fitting RGP lenses after RK. They found that efficient base curve selection using axial topography maps was achieved by selecting a base curve equal to the value 3.5 mm superior to the visual axis on an axial computerized videokeratograph.[19] This simple fitting technique works well for standard spherical RGP lens designs because it approximates the average curvature near the bend of the surgical transition zone and provides a global value for initial RGP base curve selection. Similarly, standard RGP base curves after LASIK can be chosen by choosing a curvature equal to that of the inflection point in the midperipheral cornea on the axial map. This curvature should produce a lens with midperipheral corneal alignment and adequate but not excessive central pooling.

REVERSE GEOMETRY LENSES

Many postoperative corneal surgery patients who present with oblate corneal shapes are often difficult to fit with standard RGP contact lenses.

Reverse geometry lens (RGL) designs have become popular for these patients. RGLs incorporate secondary curvatures usually 3–6 D steeper than their central curvatures (Figure 10.4), but peripheral curves have been fitted up to 15 D steeper than the central posterior curve after some surgeries. These designs are commonly used postoperatively to maintain alignment along a plateau-shaped cornea, to prevent excessive tear pooling or lens bearing, and to increase fitting stability. RGLs also assist in lens centration after RK or penetrating keratoplasty, because isolated steep areas surrounding the RK optical zone or the corneal graft can cause RGP decentration over the steepest hemimeridian of the cornea. Although RGP decentration is usually not a problem after PRK, automated lamellar keratoplasty (ALK), or LASIK, RGL fitting is still beneficial to achieve better alignment along the central and midperipheral cornea. We have fit more reverse geometry lenses after ALK and LASIK than after PRK, because use of the microkeratome causes more abrupt curvature changes surrounding the corneal cap that can occasionally affect lens centration and performance (Color Plate 9).[20] Several RGL designs have been developed in the United States, some of which were originally advocated for orthokeratology, and include the following: Plateau (Menicon USA, Ltd., Clovis, CA), OK Series (Contex

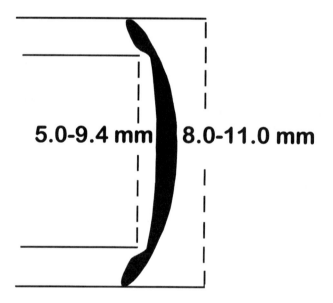

5.0-9.4 mm   **8.0-11.0 mm**

FIGURE 10.4. Cross-sectional view of a reverse geometry lens (Menicon Plateau Design, Menicon USA, Clovis, CA). (Courtesy of LB Szczotka, M Aronsky. Contact lenses after LASIK. J Am Optom Assoc 1998;69:775–784.)

Inc., Sherman Oaks, CA), RK-Bridge (Conforma, Norfolk, VA), and the NRK lens (Lancaster Contact Lens, Inc., Lancaster, PA).

The application of videokeratographic data to RGL fitting requires an understanding of peripheral shape displays and differences between axial and instantaneous reconstruction algorithms. Because instantaneous curvatures are proportional to the true local curvatures of a given peripheral corneal location, many fitters naturally assume these values are most applicable to RGL fitting, especially in the selection of secondary and peripheral lens curves. We have assessed and reported on the use of axial and instantaneous videokeratographic data to predict the required steepening in the periphery for a best fit reverse geometry RGP lens after various forms of corneal surgery that result in oblate corneal shapes.[21] We compared curvature differences (in diopters) between the base curve and the steeper secondary curve in a best fit RGL to the dioptric differences between the central and peripheral corneal curvatures from axial and instantaneous maps. Central corneal curvatures are equivalent in the axial and instantaneous displays and were recorded from the absolute central points on the topography maps. A peripheral measurement on each map was determined by positioning the cursor at the knee of the apparent surgical transition zone in each quadrant and averaging these four points. If not all of the four points were available (e.g., shadows, nose), then the remaining points were averaged. Table 10.1 displays the individual data for each patient in the study, and Table 10.2 displays the mean differences (and standard deviations) for axial, instantaneous, and contact lens curvatures. ANOVA and Tukey-Kramer post-hoc comparisons showed statistically significant differences between the central and peripheral curvatures in axial and instantaneous maps ($p < .001$) and also between the curvature differences found in instantaneous maps and the best fit contact lens ($p < .01$). There was no statistical difference between the peripheral steepening found in axial maps and the steepening required in the best fit RGP lens ($p > .05$).

Although axial and instantaneous videokeratographic data differed significantly when comparing the differences between central and peripheral corneal curvature, the axial maps were more likely to approximate the steepening required in secondary curves of reverse geometry RGP designs in postoperative corneal surgery patients with oblate corneal shapes. The fitting method should be adapted for fitting an RGL design in LASIK as follows: Select the initial base curve approximately 1 D steeper than the postoperative simulated flat K to allow for a moderate tear layer over the surgical optical zone. Occasionally, the base curve is up to 3 D steeper than the simulated flat K to allow for a smooth tear layer if significant irregularity, astigmatism, or central islands persist over the ablation zone. Some manufacturers recommend that the base curve can be selected 1 D steeper than the average keratometry reading if greater than 2 D of corneal astigmatism persists.[22] To achieve midperipheral alignment with RGL intermediate curves, begin by measuring the average midperipheral curvature at the

TABLE 10.1
Lens and Topography Data for Postsurgical Patients Fit in Reverse Geometry Lenses

Procedure	Lens Data				Axial Videokeratographic Data			Instantaneous Videokeratographic Data		
	Base Curve (D)	Secondary Curve (D)	Difference	Lens Material	Axial Central (D)	Average Axial Peripheral (D)	Difference	Instantaneous Central (D)	Average Instantaneous Peripheral (D)	Difference
Epikeratoplasty	47.5	50.4	2.9	Boston ES	45.5	48.7	3.2	45.5	51.6	6.1
Penetrating keratoplasty	44.4	48	3.6	Boston ES	46.4	50.1	3.7	46.4	52.5	6.1
ALK	41.9	45	3.1	Menicon Z	39.9	43.1	3.2	37.8	47.6	9.8
Lamellar keratoplasty	48.9	51.9	3	Menicon Z	43	46.8	3.8	43.1	49.3	6.2
Penetrating keratoplasty	42.6	45	2.4	Boston ES	42.2	45.4	3.2	42.3	48.4	6.1
Penetrating keratoplasty	43.5	48	4.5	Menicon Z	44.8	47.9	3.1	44.5	49.5	5
Penetrating keratoplasty	46.9	51.9	5	Menicon Z	42.8	46.2	3.4	43	47.2	4.2
ALK	41.1	46.1	5	Menicon Z	36.8	43.5	6.7	36.8	47.3	10.5
Epikeratoplasty, then ALK	38.3	51.9	13.6	Boston ES	34.8	44.1	9.3	34.9	51.6	16.7
Epikeratoplasty, then ALK	37.5	51.9	14.4	Boston ES	34.3	42	7.7	33.9	48.4	14.5

ALK = automated lamellar keratoplasty.
Note: Differences are between the base curve and the secondary curve of the contact lens and central data and average peripheral data on curvature maps.

TABLE 10.2
Averaged Lens and Topography Data for Patients Fit in Reverse Geometry Lenses

	Contact Lens	*Axial*	*Instantaneous*
Mean difference	5.75 D	4.73 D	8.52 D
Sample size	10	10	10
Standard deviation	4.44 D	2.28 D	4.22 D
Range	2.4–14.4 D	3.1–9.3 D	4.2–16.7 D

Note: Mean differences are between the base curve and the secondary curve of the contact lens and central data and average peripheral data on curvature maps.

knee of the transition zone on the axial topography map. This measurement is facilitated by moving the interactive cursor on topography instruments to different quadrants on the bend of the surgical optical zone. Next, calculate the average dioptric change from the center of the map to the transitions. Select a steeper RGL secondary curve in an amount equal to or up to one-third flatter than the average change noted on the axial topography map across the transition zone. For example, if the topographic steepening is 3 D, a secondary curve 2–3 D steeper than the base curve can be ordered in the RGL. Table 10.3 provides two examples of this technique, which works well to achieve an initial lens design or to help select an RGL trial lens from a diagnostic set. Patient A (Color Plate 10) was a postoperative LASIK patient with persistent hyperopic irregular astigmatism and a best corrected spectacle acuity of 20/80, 3 months after surgery. Patient B (see Color Plate 7) was a postoperative ALK patient with secondary astigmatic keratotomy enhancements with persistent undercorrection and mild irregular astigmatism 6 months after surgery.

CORNEAL CONTOUR ASSESSMENT AND RIGID GAS-PERMEABLE
LENS DIAMETER SELECTION

Overall diameter selection after LASIK often requires larger lenses than typically used for normal eyes to vault the flap and surgical optical zone. Common diameters range from 9.2 to 10.5 mm, with optical zones ranging 1–4 mm smaller than the overall diameter, depending on the surgical optical zone and lens design. The posterior contact lens optical zone should vault the LASIK ablation zone; therefore, an objective topographic measurement would be beneficial in the early design of an RGP lens.

Axial and instantaneous curvature maps vary significantly in the depiction of the apparent surgical optical zones after refractive surgery. Instantaneous maps depict a more accurate corneal shape, which is better correlated to slit-lamp observations and RGP fluorescein patterns; however,

TABLE 10.3
Examples of Reverse Geometry Lens-Fitting Techniques

	Patient A	*Patient B*
Axial topography data	Color Plate 10	Color Plate 11
Central curvature	37.73 D	37.87 D
Simulated flat K	39.42 D	38.13 D
Simulated steep K	39.84 D	39.06 D
Peripheral transition curves		
Superior	Missing	Missing
Temporal	41.36 D	44 D
Inferior	Missing	Missing
Nasal	42 D	43.98 D
Average	41.68 D	44.99 D
Central-peripheral difference	3.95 D	7.03 D
RGL parameters		
Base curve (BC)	8.45 mm (39.87 D)	8.2 mm (41.12 D)
Diameter	9.8 mm	10 mm
Optical zone	8.2 mm	8 mm
Secondary curve (SC)	7.9 mm (42.62 D)/ 0.4 mm width	7.32 mm (46 D)/ 0.4 mm width
Tertiary curve	9.9 mm/0.2 mm width	8.82 mm/0.3 mm width
Peripheral curve	11.5 mm/0.2 mm width	11.5 mm/0.3 mm width
Power	–0.50 D	–6 D
BC-SC difference	2.75 D	4.88 D

K = keratometry reading; RGL = reverse geometry lens.

elevation maps display data even differently from curvature maps. Most elevation maps depict relative height differences from a reference sphere in which reds or warmer colors usually denote higher elevation values and blues or cooler colors denote areas of the cornea that are lower than the specified reference sphere. Once elevation maps become familiar to the user, they are useful in predicting the appearance of what an RGP fluorescein pattern may look like after LASIK (or any cornea) without interpreting curvature maps (Color Plate 11). The high (red) areas will always displace fluorescein and the low (blue) areas will always pool fluorescein. This is in contrast to curvature maps, in which both steep (red) and flat (blue) areas may either displace or pool fluorescein, depending on the corneal location.[23]

Elevation maps are useful in the selection of RGP optical zone sizes after LASIK. Surgical optical zones are difficult to measure objectively after

LASIK, and elevation maps are one method that can help predict the best fit RGP lens and fluorescein pattern. For example, the size of the RGP optical zone can be targeted to vault the surgical optical zone, as noted on the elevation map. Lens optical zones are typically between 6 and 8 mm and are large enough to vault most LASIK optical zones that range from 4.5–6.0 mm.[2,3,7] The lens optical zone must also be large enough to provide full pupillary coverage in dim illumination to prevent glare and halos that many patients originally sought to correct by pursuing rigid lenses. Sufficiently large lens optical zone sizes can only prevent the type of glare caused by small optical zones that intersect the entrance pupil. Glare caused by interface haze cannot by corrected with RGP lenses, and small lens optical zones may additionally contribute to symptoms of glare or halos in these patients.

RIGID GAS-PERMEABLE LENS DESIGN SELECTION
FOR OBLATE CORNEAL SHAPES

The choice of which RGP design to use after LASIK, PRK, or ALK depends on a combination of fitter preferences, the corneal contour, patient comfort, and previous RGP lens performance. There may not be one correct design selection, and often many designs are physiologically and visually acceptable.

My guidelines for choosing standard or reverse geometry RGP design are listed in Table 10.4. Standard RGP designs with traditional, flatter secondary and peripheral curve systems work well on symmetric corneas with no isolated areas of abrupt corneal contour changes surrounding the flap or

TABLE 10.4
Rigid Gas-Permeable Lens (RGP) Design Selection for Oblate Corneal Shapes

Standard RGP design
    Symmetric OZ
    No isolated steep area surrounding OZ
    High corneal eccentricity (e >0.55)
    Smooth/unaltered corneal periphery
      (LASIK, photorefractive keratectomy, ALK)
Reverse geometry lens design
    Isolated steep area/abrupt changes surrounding surgical OZ
    RGP decentration with standard designs
    Altered corneal periphery (i.e., RK)
    Low corneal eccentricity (e <0.55)
    Need for better alignment, even FL pattern

ALK = automated lamellar keratoplasty; FL = fluorescein; OZ = optical zone; RK = radial keratotomy.

surgical optical zone. These designs work well most often in uncomplicated LASIK or PRK and when the patient is seeking contact lens correction
for residual, regular under- or overcorrection.

Standard lens designs also work well on eyes that had higher than
average preoperative corneal eccentricity (e >0.55). The average cornea has
an eccentricity of approximately e = 0.55. On an eye with rapid peripheral
flattening (e.g., e = 0.75), the secondary and peripheral curve systems of a
standard RGP design on an ablated cornea may be sufficient to allow satisfactory midperipheral corneal alignment. Conversely, on an eye with a low
preoperative corneal eccentricity (e.g., e = 0.3), the corneal periphery
approaches that of a sphere, and after ablation of the central cornea, a large
disparity may exist between the peripheral corneal and RGP curvatures if
the lens has been fit appropriately to the central cornea. Eyes with low preoperative corneal eccentricities often require an RGL design for best performance. Reverse geometry designs also work best on corneas with abrupt
contour changes surrounding the surgical optical zone that may encourage
decentration of standard lens designs, and on eyes with surgically altered
corneal peripheries as in RK.

Pearl:
Corneas with high preprocedure eccentricity do well with standard
designs. Low preprocedure corneal eccentricity does better with a reverse
geometry lens.

I rarely use aspheric designs on oblate corneal shapes, although the
successful use of a low eccentricity lens design (Boston Envision [Polymer
Technology/Bausch & Lomb, Rochester, New York]) after PRK has been
reported in the literature.[13] High eccentricity RGP lens designs flatten
excessively in the lens periphery and are counterproductive to achieving
better midperipheral corneal alignment on oblate corneal shapes. Additionally, if an aspheric lens decenters, visual acuity can be compromised from
unanticipated power changes positioned over the entrance pupil.

PHYSIOLOGIC FACTORS INFLUENCING CONTACT LENS FITTING

Corneal wound healing responses are less of a concern after LASIK than
after RK or PRK. The shift to an intrastromal ablation eliminates the epithelial healing phase and the epithelial cell or stromal keratocyte interac-
tions seen in PRK that result in subepithelial haze and regression.[24]
Potential physiologic changes that may affect contact lens wear after LASIK
include an uneven tear film due to an irregular corneal surface, temporary
loss of sensory innervation from severed corneal nerves, and transient corneal thickness changes.[3] One of LASIK's safety concerns is its effect on the
corneal endothelium because of the close proximity and secondary effect of
acoustic shock waves to the posterior cornea.[8,24] Most studies report that

LASIK does not cause any damage to the central corneal endothelium up to 12 months after surgery.[24-26] In fact, short-term postoperative improvements have been recorded in endothelial cell density and morphometric indexes that are believed to be related to postoperative discontinuation of contact lens use. Long-term studies on the integrity of the endothelium after LASIK are timely and warranted.

The additional effect of contact lens wear may add stress to an already compromised cornea. To preserve the remaining flap, stromal, and endothelial integrity, RGP lenses with moderate to high oxygen transmissibility should be prescribed when worn full time. A typical postoperative LASIK contact lens power of –3.00 D and a center thickness of approximately 0.12 mm should have, at minimum, a Dk value greater than 40 to achieve an oxygen transmissibility (Dk/L) sufficient for the eye's respiratory needs.[27] Material stability is important for efficient manufacturing and minimal on-eye flexure, especially in reverse curve designs. New high-Dk RGP polymers that are stable enough to be manufactured in thin lens designs are recommended.

Summary

Although patients may be apprehensive to pursue contact lens fitting after elective refractive surgery, the principles outlined here turn a potentially difficult fitting into a teachable science. If managed appropriately, the patients should enjoy unlimited years of clear vision and successful contact lens wear.

References

1. Waring GO III, Lynn MJ, McDonnell PJ, et al. Results of the prospective evaluation of radial keratotomy (PERK) study 10 years after surgery. Arch Ophthalmol 1994;112:1298–1308.

2. Danasoury MA, Waring GO, El-Maghraby AE, Mehrez K. Excimer laser in situ keratomileusis to correct compound myopic astigmatism. J Refract Surg 1997;13:511–520.

3. Perez-Santonja JJ, Bellot J, Claramonte P, et al. Laser in situ keratomileusis to correct high myopia. J Cataract Refact Surg 1997;23:372–385.

4. MacRae S, Rich L, Phillips D, Bedrossian R. Diurnal variation in vision after radial keratotomy. Am J Ophthalmol 1989;107:262–267.

5. McDonnell PJ, Caroline PJ, Salz J. Irregular astigmatism after radial and astigmatic keratotomy. Am J Ophthalmol 1989;107:42–46.

6. Mulhern MM, Foley-Nolan A, O'Keefe M, Condon P. Topographical analysis of ablation centration after excimer laser photorefractive keratectomy and laser in situ keratomileusis for high myopia. J Cataract Refract Surg 1997;23: 488–494.

7. Tsai RJ. Laser in situ keratomileusis for myopia of –2 to –25 diopters. J Refract Surg 1997;13:S427–S429.

8. Pallilkaris I, Siganos D. Laser in situ keratomileusis to treat myopia: early experience. J Cataract Refact Surg 1997;23:39–49.

9. Wang Z, Chen J, Yang B. Comparison of laser in situ keratomileusis and photorefractive keratectomy to correct myopia from –1.25 to –6.00 diopters. J Refact Surg 1997;13:528–534.

10. Srur M, Dattas D. The use of disposable contact lenses as therapeutic lenses. CLAO J 1997;23:40–42.

11. Weiner B. How and when to prescribe bandage contact lenses. Rev Optom 1996;133:38–42.

12. Kanellopoulos AJ, Pallikaris IG, Donnenfeld ED, et al. Comparison of corneal sensation following photorefractive keratectomy and laser in situ keratomileusis. J Cataract Refact Surg 1997;23:34–38.

13. Shipper I, Businger U, Psarrer R. Fitting contact lenses after excimer laser photorefractive keratectomy for myopia. CLAO J 1995;21:281–284.

14. Schivitz IA, Arrowsmith PN, Russell BM. Contact lenses in the treatment of patients with overcorrected radial keratotomy. Ophthalmology 1987;94:899–903.

15. Lee AM, Kastl PR. Rigid gas permeable contact lens fitting after radial keratotomy. CLAO J 1998;24:33–35.

16. Campbell MD, Caroline P. A unique technique for fitting post RK patient. Contact Lens Spect 1994;12:56.

17. Chan J, Burger D. The use of peripheral corneal measurements for fitting an RK/PRK patient. Optom Vis Sci 1996;73(12S):235.

18. Roberts C. Comparison of characteristic corneal topography patterns following radial keratotomy using two reconstruction algorithms. Invest Ophthalmol Vis Sci 1997;38:S921.

19. McDonnell PJ, Garbus JJ, Caroline P, Yoshinaga PD. Computerized analysis of corneal topography as an aid in fitting contact lenses after radial keratotomy. Ophthalmol Surg 1992;23:55–59.

20. Edwards KH, Hough DA, Kersley HJ. Designing rigid lenses for the post PRK eye. Optom Vis Sci 1995;72(12S):13.

21. Aronsky MA, Aggarwal T, Reinhart WJ, Szczotka LB. Application of videokeratographic data for fitting reverse geometry contact lenses in post-corneal surgery patients. Invest Ophthalmol Vis Sci 1998;39S:1545.

22. Menicon Plateau Fitting Guide, Menicon U.S.A., Clovis, CA, 1996.

23. Szczotka LB, Lebow K. Corneal Topography for Contact Lens Fitting. Optometry Today 1998;6(6):38–46.

24. Kent DG, Solomon KD, Peng Q, et al. Effect of surface photorefractive and laser in situ keratomileusis on the corneal endothelium. J Cataract Refact Surg 1997;23:386–397.

25. Perez-Santonja JJ, Sakla HF, Gobbi F, Alio JL. Corneal endothelial changes after laser in situ keratomileusis. J Cataract Refract Surg 1997;23:177–183.

26. Perez-Santonja JJ, Sakla HF, Alio JL. Evaluation of endothelial cell changes 1 year after excimer laser in situ keratomileusis. Arch Ophthalmol 1997;115: 841–846.
27. Mizutani Y, Matsutaka H, Takemoto N. The effect of anoxia on the human cornea. Acta Soc Ophthalmol Jpn 1987;9:644–649.

CHAPTER 11

Future Techniques and Investigational Procedures

Joseph P. Shovlin, Michael R. Boland, Paul M. Karpecki, Steven H. Linn, and Michael D. DePaolis

Concerns and limitations in corneal shaping, both anatomic and functional, have forced investigators to explore innovative extraocular and intraocular techniques to treat refractive errors. In our quest to find the very best procedure for every refractive anomaly, we have investigated several new frontiers and some familiar procedures from the past with renewed interest. Concerns in existing surgical procedures, especially surface area and thickness volume techniques, have spurred investigators to find procedures with increased safety profiles that are reversible, stable, and predictable.[1–3]

Several investigational procedures currently under way, as well as some future concepts, are reviewed in this chapter, including linking systems for excimer ablation procedures, the use of nonexcimer lasers, intraocular lenses for phakic patients with high refractive errors, intracorneal implants, and experimental procedures for presbyopia. Where appropriate and when they exist, investigational results and future direction are highlighted.

Linking Systems for Excimer Ablation

TOPOGRAPHY-CONTROLLED ABLATION

New programs that use the excimer laser to integrate corneal topography into ablation patterns are being developed. The Visx Cap Method for the Staar S2 System (Visx, Santa Clara, CA) allows surgeons to vary ablation location, depth, shape, and size using a proprietary beam-shaping module to narrow and redirect the seven-beam scanning array of the Staar S2. This provides smooth, virtually seamless ablations. The company has used several different topographers to date.

Special attention has been directed toward treating irregular corneas, such as those with keratoconus, postpenetrating keratoplasty, decentered ablations, central islands, and inferior corneal steepening. Using topography ablation–planning software, practitioners can visualize the intended ablation ahead of time and plan programs for further refinement.

WAVE FRONT TECHNOLOGY

The Bausch and Lomb/Chiron Technolas 217 laser (Chiron, Claremont, CA) uses a 2-mm spot size to ablate a smooth surface on the cornea and is ergonomically designed specifically for LASIK. Bausch and Lomb recently purchased Orbtek (Salt Lake City), which manufactures the Orbscan II Corneal topography unit. Orbtek topography provides additional information, such as elevation of the front and back surfaces of the cornea, corneal thickness, and topography (Figure 11.1).[2] By combining the Orbscan with ultrasound to determine axial length and lens thickness, a simulation of the retinal point spread function (PSF) can be determined. Orbtek has created a simulated measurement technique called *wavefront ablation vision enhancement*

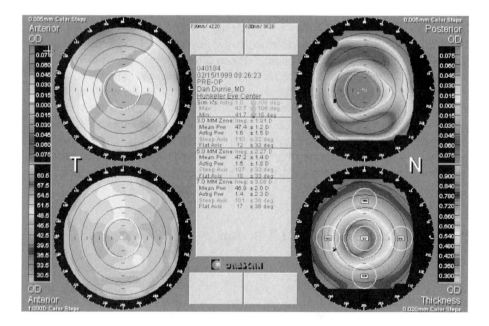

FIGURE 11.1. Orbtek topography shows various features of a cornea following photorefractive keratectomy retreatment with posterior surface ectasia. Elevation of the front surface of the cornea (*top left map*), elevation of the back surface of the cornea (*top right map*), corneal thickness (*bottom right*), and topography (*bottom left*) are shown. (OD = right eye.)

(WAVE). Rather than relying solely on corneal measurements, WAVE is designed to treat the visual system by targeting idealistic postoperative topography with optic PSF. Reverse ray tracing is then applied to create patterns involving all aspects of the visual system, from corneal Orbscan measurements, to lens index and thickness, to retinal spacing. The WAVE system is still experimental and has yet to begin human clinical trials.

Custom Cornea

Beyond topography guided ablation, a device called *Custom Cornea*, developed by Autonomous Technology Inc., a subsidiary of Summit Technology Inc. (Waltham, MA), will soon be introduced. Last year, Autonomous became the third laser company to receive FDA approval. The LADAR-Vision excimer laser (Autonomous Technology Inc., Orlando, FL) was approved for treatment of myopia up to 10 D and astigmatism up to 4 D. The laser uses a 0.8- to 0.1-mm small spot beam and a National Aeronautics and Space Administration (NASA)–developed eye tracker. Software-controlled ablation algorithms are used to create shot patterns that direct each of the thousands of individual pulses to a predetermined location. This allows a smoother overlapping pattern and the potential to place the spots where desired for optimal vision results. The LADARVision eye-tracker checks the position of the eye 4,000 times per second and then adjusts the position of the laser pulse. This system can compensate for the smallest eye movements, including saccades.

Autonomous' most exciting development may be the custom cornea project. It uses a proprietary wavefront sensor to actually measure the total aberrations of the eye. A laser pulse travels through the cornea, lens, media, and retina. Returning retinal waves are measured. The custom cornea measurement device currently used on patients clearly shows that, when considering the entire visual system from cornea to retina, patients with above-average vision have significantly fewer aberrations.[2] This technology and measurement of aberrations and their exact location, combined with the eye tracker technology of LADARVision, may have more patients seeing 20/10.

Biomask Technology

Biomask technology uses, with the excimer laser, a liquid collagen–derived material that has been cross-linked. It serves as spackle as it ablates at the same approximate rate as corneal tissue. Although this procedure's initial indications are slated for treating those with irregular corneal surfaces, the technology may transfer well to treating various refractive errors, especially overcorrections after initial laser surgery.

The principle behind this technology is to apply the material onto the cornea, then mold it to solidify with a significantly steeper cornea surface. Ablation is then carried out based on the results desired. The technique is currently used as a smoothing procedure when the cornea has opacity or irregularity. As the laser ablates the mask, it trims the steeper areas of the cornea that break through first. During this process, the curvature of the front of the mask is transferred to the cornea. Patients with neovascularization should be excluded from having this procedure performed due to potential for significant bleeding during the procedure. Surgeons should be extremely careful not to tilt the contact lens when covering the Biomask.

Epithelial Autofluorescence

Investigators are also studying how epithelial autofluorescence can be used to guide transepithelial ablation to treat mild overcorrections after photorefractive keratectomy (PRK) or LASIK. This technique can be used without raising the flap in LASIK patients.

New Flap Makers

As lamellar surgery continues to evolve, the role of instrumentation to create a flap becomes increasingly more important. Most perioperative complications encountered in this type of surgery relate to the making of the flap. New technology in making a flap has shifted from standard microkeratomes (conventional and disposable) to other ways to dissect the stroma.

Water Jet Technology

Automated water jet technology allows surgeons to safely create a smooth flap using a water beam. Flap diameters range from 6–11 mm. Current instruments are made by two manufacturers, the Medjet (Alcon, Fort Worth, TX) and the Visijet Hydrokeratome (Princeton, NJ).

Laser

Lasers can make adjustable flaps ranging in diameter up to 10 mm. The IntraLase Femtosecond Laser (University of Heidelberg, Heidelberg, Germany) and the Novatec Laser Microkeratome (Carlsbad, CA) are currently under investigation (see the section Ultrafast Lasers for a full description of this technology).

In addition to creating flaps, the Novatec Laser creates intrastromal bubbles for refractive effects using transmissive wavelength lasers.

Investigational Nonexcimer Lasers

Laser Thermal Keratoplasty

Laser thermal keratoplasty (LTK) is a process that uses controlled quantities of thermal energy to heat the cornea, thereby shortening the collagen fibers and altering corneal curvature. The pulsed holmium:yttrium aluminum garnet (Ho:YAG) at a wavelength of 2.06–2.15 µm has become the laser of choice for LTK; with a penetration depth of 480–530 µm, it allows for stromal heating with minimal adjacent tissue damage.[4] The conic temperature profile administered by this laser offers more pronounced collagen shrinkage anteriorly, producing more effective refractive results and improved stability over time.[1] A noncontact device by Sunrise Technologies (Fremont, CA) has proven to be the best instrument for this thermal delivery system with a very promising future for the surgical correction of both hyperopia and presbyopia (Figure 11.2).

A slit-lamp delivery system is used for LTK, delivering up to 8 spots in the corneal midperiphery, with 2 concentric rings at approximately 6 and 7 mm, respectively. Overcorrections after PRK and LASIK have been treated successfully using only one concentric ring. A lid speculum is used after the first anesthetic drop is administered. Once corneal hydration is properly controlled and good fixation is present, the pulses are delivered at a 5-Hz pulse repetition frequency with pulse energy ranging from 208–242 mJ.[3]

Seth E. Murphy, O.D.
Doctor of Optometry

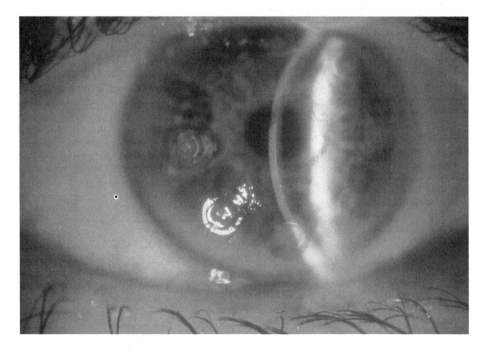

FIGURE 11.2. Thermal delivery systems work by shrinking collagen to steepen the cornea. Note the circular pattern to the treatment applied to the cornea.

Topical antibiotic and nonsteroidal anti-inflammatory agents are used post-operatively four times a day until the epithelium heals.

Preliminary studies in the United States, Germany, and Canada have concluded that LTK is a safe and effective procedure with very low rates of complication not only for hyperopia up to 2.5 D, but for presbyopia as well. Transient myopic shift in the first month postoperatively has been widely reported, but results have been very stable from that point on. Results from a phase 3 FDA study of safety and efficacy of the Sunrise Technologies Inc. (Fremont, CA) Sun 1000 Corneal Shaping Ho:YAG laser for LTK treatment of hyperopia have exceeded FDA targets.[3] Although early studies for astigmatic correction with the contact LTK system by Summit Technologies were discontinued, the noncontact device has a much brighter future and will be investigated as the trials continue.

A study analyzing changes in corneal curvature induced by LTK was conducted at Cullen Eye Institute (Baylor University, Houston, TX). Computerized videokeratography was measured preoperatively and at day 1, 1 month, 3 months, and 12 months postoperatively. Curvature was measured at the 1-, 3-, 5-, and 7-mm zones. The study concluded that peripheral corneal flattening and central corneal steepening were produced by noncontact Ho:YAG LTK, with a two-ring treatment causing the greatest curvature change.[5]

Ideal candidates are at least 40 years of age, have less than 1 D of astigmatism, have either mild to moderate hyperopia or emmetropia, and desire presbyopic correction (monovision). Age 40 years is the minimum age, because the thermal effect on collagen is somewhat age-dependent. Once the procedure is completed, patients experience their correction immediately, because they are slightly overcorrected at first. One procedure takes approximately 2.4 seconds of laser time and is technically quite simple to perform.[5] Because the 6-mm concentric treatment ring is outside the visual axis, glare and halos are uncommon with LTK.

LTK has shown excellent potential for treatment of hyperopia, presbyopia, and even for overcorrected PRK and LASIK. As more studies are completed, parameters that maximize predictability, efficacy, and stability should be found. In clinical trials, approximately 80% of patients are within 0.5 D of emmetropia, no patient has lost best corrected acuity, and regression has been minimal.[1,4,5]

RADIOFREQUENCY KERATOPLASTY

Radiofrequency keratoplasty is an investigational procedure for reducing or eliminating hyperopia. The procedure reshapes the cornea by delivering high frequency radio waves through a probe inserted into the superficial cornea. The device is called the *Refractec* (Refractec Co., Irvine, CA) and is currently under a multicenter prospective clinical trial. Early results from phase 3 trials and more extensive international trials indicate that visual stability, an early potential concern, should not be a problem. Investigators have found that with thermal lesions applied to the cornea, long-term stability, rather than safety, becomes an issue. All 2-year studies have shown 100% of the eyes to be stable between 1 and 2 years, with no cases of best corrected vision loss or other significant corneal complications.[6]

GEL INJECTION ADJUSTABLE KERATOPLASTY

Gel injection adjustable keratoplasty (GIAK) requires the injection of a gel material into a carefully dissected pocket of the stroma to change the anterior corneal curvature irreversibly. GIAK is a relatively simple, inexpensive procedure that simultaneously corrects myopia and astigmatism. Gabriel Simon developed GIAK in 1985.[1] Initial studies used a soft intracorneal ring. Later, various materials were used and found to provide the advantages of adjustability and ease of manipulation. The current material used is polyethylene oxide.[1] Long-term biocompatibility has been demonstrated.

The procedure is easily performed using topical anesthetic. A diamond knife is set at 80% thickness, and a radial incision is made shorter than 1 mm in length. A helicoid spatula is used to make a 360 degree intrastromal channel at the depth of the radial incision. The exact amount of gel required is injected into the channel tract in small aliquots. The amount depends on the desired refractive effect and is determined by monitoring the intraoperative curvature of the anterior cornea.[1]

Human studies began in 1996 in eyes without sight, and sighted eye studies are now under way. Several unresolved issues exist. Accurate tables are not available to dictate operative parameters, and the material injected is opaque in the stroma, requiring a sufficiently large clear zone of the cornea.[1] A unique feature is the adjustability of this technique, which theoretically allows for titration of refractive error at any later date. There appears to be little, if any, risk of scarring and persistent haze.

ULTRAFAST LASERS

According to the Femto Group at the University of Heidelberg, therapeutic laser applications in today's medicine are primarily based on a photoablative interaction process between the laser radiation and the tissue. Such medical lasers are operated down to pulse widths in the range of nanoseconds. One of the problems with such thermal lasers is that the zones of interaction are poorly localized because of heat diffusion in the tissue. By using very short, high-intensity laser pulses in the range of picoseconds or femtoseconds, a different interaction mechanism occurs. This interaction is a plasma-mediated ablation.[7] In this type of laser tissue interaction, microplasma and tissue removal are created by a combination of multiphoton absorption and an avalanche-like ionization process. This is termed *laser-induced optic breakdown*. The Femto Group reports that there are usually no thermal side effects from such a procedure because interaction times are shorter than the time for thermal diffusion.

The majority of today's refractive surgery techniques to correct myopia typically involve removing tissue to alter corneal curvature, as in excimer laser PRK and LASIK. In contrast, with ultraviolet laser photoablation, as with the excimer laser (wavelength, 193 nm), ultrashort laser pulses that operate at infrared wavelengths can be focused inside a transparent media, such as the cornea, with proper focusing geometries. Ultrafast lasers, such as the picosecond and femtosecond lasers, using high powered pulses of infrared laser light, can be focused at a specified depth within the transparent cornea.[8] Absorption of the laser energy creates a microplasma, leading to increased pressure and temperature. At this site, shock or stress waves are created by the expansion of the microplasma, generating a cavitation bubble (Figure 11.3).

These precise foci of laser pulses can be directed in the form of a spiral placed at a certain depth, with pulses given until a bed of overlapping cavitation bubbles is created. The tissue in the small volume where the cavitation bubbles were created is destroyed as the bubbles collapse. This laser spiraling pattern can be created at two specified depths with a given tissue thickness between the cavitation bubble beds, creating a lenticule of corneal tissue. At the edges of the bed(s), a series of decreasing depth laser pulses in a ring pattern can virtually cut the tissue anteriorly to the corneal surface. This ability to cut laterally to make a slice inside the cornea, com-

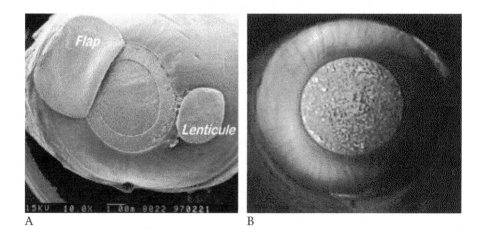

A   B

FIGURE 11.3. **(A)** Scanning electron microscopy of an eye after performing femtosecond intrastromal keratomileusis procedure. **(B)** View through the surgical microscope during intrastromal photorefractive keratectomy. Light is reflected at tiny bubbles generated by plasma. (Courtesy of Femto Group, University of Heidelberg, Heidelberg, Germany.)

bined with the ability to cut anteriorly toward the corneal surface, provides a nonmechanic way to create a LASIK flap and to remove tissue by the formation of a lenticule of corneal stroma. The lenticule can be removed with surgical forceps.

Ultrafast lasers can cut a flap for LASIK by creating a bed at a given depth—for example, 160 mm—and with a specified diameter. The same laser, focused in a ring pattern, can cut up to the corneal surface around the diameter of the cavitation bed at continuously decreasing depths. The laser leaves a hinge of designated width like a corneal flap created by a microkeratome. This procedure has been tested on human eyes by Krueger et al. using a neodymium-doped yttrium-lithium-fluoride (Nd:YLF) picosecond laser at 1,053 nm to create a 6-mm flap, combined with an excimer laser to perform LASIK. Krueger et al. have also used the picosecond laser for laser keratomileusis, creating an intrastromal lenticule with two cavitation bubble beds at two different depths. A faster laser, the femtosecond laser, should allow for larger optic zone diameter than the picosecond laser, up to 9 mm according to the Femto Group, and can create a curved anterior bed of cavitation bubbles when cutting a lenticule. A lenticule of varying thickness can be cut to achieve different levels of corneal flattening to correct various levels of myopia (Figure 11.4).

Researchers are continuing the study of ultrafast lasers and their medical and ophthalmologic applications. In ophthalmic surgery, techniques are being evaluated to remove tissue by layered intrastromal photoablation. This technique, by creating several disc-like layers of cavitation shock wave photodisruption, creates an intrastromal space. This space closes as the cavitation bubbles collapse, flattening the corneal curvature. This pro-

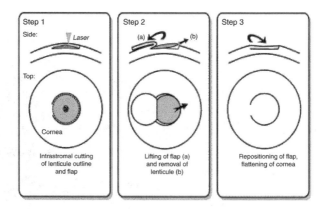

FIGURE 11.4. Three steps in completing a corneal flap to correct various degrees of myopia (see text).

cedure is called *intrastromal keratectomy.* According to the Femto Group, animal studies of this procedure showed corneal clarity returned within 3 days of the procedure without significant corneal haze (Figure 11.5).[7]

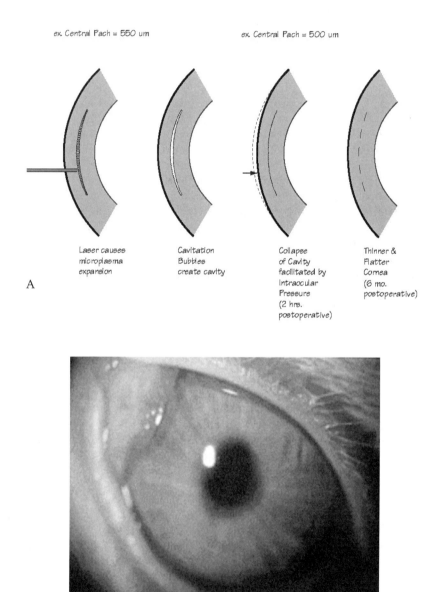

FIGURE 11.5. Femtosecond keratomileusis (**A**) with corneal transparency completely returned 1 week postoperatively (**B**). (Courtesy of the Femto Group, University of Heidelberg, Heidelberg, Germany.)

Phakic Intraocular Lenses

Several new phakic intraocular lenses for the correction of ametropia are under investigation. The concept of phakic intraocular lenses originated in the 1950s, when myopic anterior chamber lenses were designed and implanted by Strampelli, Barraquer, Danheim, and Choyce.[1,9] Fechner et al. revived this concept by developing an iris-fixated lens. Joly et al. developed an angle-supported phakic intraocular lens derived from the Kelman Multiflex lens.[1] In 1991, the Moscow Research Institute of Eye Microsurgery reported on the use of a phakic posterior chamber lens to correct high myopia.[9] Since then, phakic intraocular lenses have received increased attention as a means of correcting high ametropia.[1]

Lenses are classified by their anatomic position within the eye. Each of the currently tested designs has a unique configuration involving both the haptics and the optic portion of the lens. Currently, at least three different types of phakic intraocular lenses are under investigation at the FDA. Each offers unique advantages but poses distinct concerns.[1,9] Potential advantages exist over corneal procedures used for refractive surgery, including the potential to adjust and reverse the effects by removing the lens whenever necessary. In addition, the surgical techniques used are familiar to most ophthalmic surgeons; therefore, surgeons do not have to learn new procedures or purchase new equipment required in other refractive techniques.[1] Higher refractive errors are easily corrected while maintaining corneal asphericity, as compared to corneal refractive procedures that have a practical limit of 12–15 D depending on patient profile (corneal thickness, curvature, and pupil size). The assumption is based on a required post-LASIK posterior lamellar thickness of 225–250 μm; the post-PRK requirement is 350 μm.[1]

Pearl:
Phakic intraocular lasers allow corneal asphericity to remain intact while correcting higher refractive errors.

Despite the listed benefits of intraocular surgery, several disadvantages and concerns exist. Foremost is the risk of intraocular surgery with all of the attendant complications. Apart from the known risks of intraocular surgery (infection, cystoid macular edema, glaucoma, cataracts, and retinal detachment), surgeons performing these procedures must also consider the added difficulties in determining the lens power calculations that eyes with extreme refractive errors present.[1,9,10] Holladays' formula, taking into account anterior chamber depth and overall length of the eye, as well as other formulas that are currently available, may aid significantly in determining lens power.

ANTERIOR CHAMBER LENSES

Anterior chamber lenses are configured to position in front of the iris and are stabilized generally by the haptics that anchor in the angle. Phacodonesis has been a problem with some first-generation designs. Corneal decompensation after significant insult to corneal endothelium is another possible complication. Uveitis-glaucoma-hyphema syndromes were once again part of the postoperative complication list. First-generation lenses included the Baikoff angle-supported lens, the Momose spider lens and the Worst Iris Claw Lens.

The Baikoff anterior chamber multiflex style lens (Bausch & Lomb NuVita/Domilens, Rochester, NY) (Figure 11.6) and the 6-µm heparin-coated Phakic 6 intraocular lens (IOL) (Ophthalmic Innovations International, Claremont, CA) are two noniris-fixed anterior chamber lenses currently being investigated in clinical trials monitored by the FDA. The Artisan myopic lens (Ophtec USA, Boca Raton, FL) designed by Worst is an anterior chamber lens attached to the iris. The lens is fixated by iris capture in the two haptics.

Baikoff Anterior Chamber Multiflex Style Lens

Modification of the successful polymethylmethacrylate Kelman four-point fixation angle-supported lens by Baikoff (Lyon, France) (1986) led to the possibility of implanting a phakic intraocular lens to maintain accommodation in patients with high refractive errors. The Baikoff lens design was familiar to surgeons making it and was perhaps the easiest of the first-generation lenses

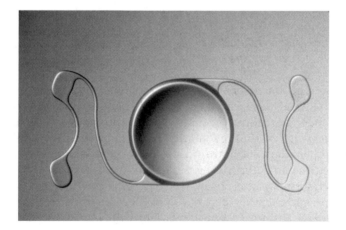

FIGURE 11.6. Bausch & Lomb's newly redesigned NuVita anterior chamber phakic intraocular lens. (Courtesy of Bausch & Lomb, Lyon, France.)

to insert and remove if necessary.[1] The early design (Domilens model ZB) produced progressive endothelial cell loss, which often began in the midperiphery of the cornea over the edge of the lens optic. The problem, caused by excessive lens vaulting and edge thickness, necessitated explantation rates of over 50%.[1,10] Difficulty in accurately sizing the lens to the anterior chamber diameter led to lens rotation if the lens was too small or to ocular tenderness, iris retraction, and pupil ovalization if it was too large.[1,11] Additional concerns with this lens included small optic zone size, required incision size, complaints of glare or halos, and long-term subclinical inflammation. Focal iris atrophy and angle damage have also been reported.[10]

Several postsurveillance studies have been published. Baikoff has reported 3-year follow-up results of the ZB5M multicenter study in France. Predictability in calculating lens power was acceptable, with more than 80% of the patients falling within ± 1 D of emmetropia. The rate of endothelial cell loss at 3 years was 6%.[3] To date, none of the patients has had a lens removed secondary to endothelial cell loss or damage. Fewer than 5% have ovalization of the pupil. The most troubling complaint is a 23% reporting rate of nocturnal halos.[1]

Kaufman reported on 10 eyes implanted with the Baikoff ZB5M lens that had high myopia. He found no significant endothelial cell loss in the early postoperative follow-up. Patients uniformly complained of glare and halos, and pupil ovalization resulted in a discontinuation of the FDA study of this model.[1,9,10] Marinho et al. found late complications consisting of cataracts and retinal detachment in 0.5% of patients who were implanted with the ZB5M lens.[10]

Decreasing the angle of the IOL shoulder and optic thickness appears to have lessened the problem of endothelial cell loss in the newer lens (Bausch & Lomb/NuVita MA20). This third-generation version is now being manufactured with an improved footplate design to decrease pupil ovalization and provide for better natural lens clearance. The peripheral detail (antiglare) treatment has been used to modify the larger 5.0-mm optic edge and minimize glare and halos. Additionally, a redesign of the haptics to make them more flexible has eliminated iris retraction, which had caused pupil ovalization (Figure 11.7).

The lens is available in powers from 7–20 D of myopia. This design can be inserted through a temporal clear corneal or scleral incision using standard surgical techniques. Care must be taken to avoid contact with the crystalline lens. Alleman, using ultrasound biomicroscopy to determine safe implantation selection, concluded that an anterior chamber depth should measure 2.3 mm or larger for safe implantation of this lens.[12]

Phakic 6 Intraocular Lens

The Phakic 6 IOL is a heparin surface anterior chamber lens modified by Galen and manufactured by Ophthalmic Innovations International (Claremont, CA). The heparin coating is believed to reduce the risk of infection

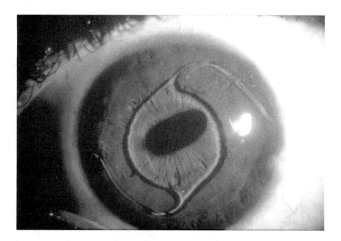

FIGURE 11.7. Iris contracture causing pupil ovalization owing to a poorly fitted anterior chamber phakic intraocular lens. (Courtesy of Herbert Kaufman, MD, LSU Eye Center, New Orleans, LA.)

and chronic inflammation. The 6-mm optic minimizes glare and halos. Endothelial and iris contact is avoided by a flexible design that offers almost no resistance and minimizes ovalization. The lens is designed to correct for myopia with a power range of 5–25 D and hyperopia with a power range of 2–10 D. Astigmatism is corrected by corneal incision placement (a form of astigmatic keratotomy) as the lens is inserted. Most, if not all, cataract surgeons place an incision along the steeper meridian when significant corneal astigmatism is present.

Few studies assess the safety and efficacy of the Phakic 6 IOL. Clinical trials are soon to be under way at the FDA. A recent Investigational Device Exemption has been granted by the FDA. In a small series, Hirschman reports no primary removals and enhanced best corrected visual acuity in many of the patients who were implanted.[10]

Worst-Fechner Artisan Iris Claw Lens

The Iris Claw phakic lens design has received much support from the European ophthalmic community, in which Worst and Fechner have implanted these lenses successfully for more than 15 years. The Artisan lens attaches to the peripheral iris with two claws (Figure 11.8). The lens is placed away from the crystalline lens, can be centered over the pupil, and avoids the angle. Available powers range from 5–23 D of myopic correction.

Because the lens is not foldable, it does require a sutured corneal incision. Centration can be a problem, as it may reposition after initial placement. The technique of placement is somewhat more challenging, because the surgeon must fixate the lens over the pupil while tucking the peripheral

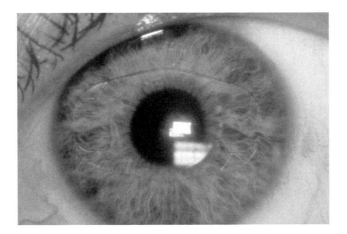

FIGURE 11.8. Worst's Artisan Iris Claw Lens corrects myopia by attaching to the peripheral iris for support.

iris into one of the claws for enclavation. A spreader is used to create a fold in the iris. To prevent pupillary block, a peripheral iridectomy is performed. Potential complications are more likely to occur from the surgical technique of implantation than from the properties of the lens itself.[1] The major postoperative concerns are chronic low-grade inflammation and long-term corneal endothelial stability. This lens design may induce a greater breakdown of the blood-aqueous barrier and induce more chronic inflammation, which may adversely affect endothelial cell counts.[1,10,13,14]

Recently published reports from Menezo et al. have found that after 3 years' follow-up of 58 eyes, 60% of eyes achieved 20/40 or better uncorrected visual acuity, and 77% of eyes gained 2 or more lines of best corrected visual acuity. The predictability was excellent because 48% and 79% of eyes were within ± 0.5 D or ± 1 D of emmetropia. No major complications were reported; however, endothelial cell loss was 17.9% at 5 years after surgery.[1] Another study has found the anterior chamber flare values were significantly higher for this design at 2-year follow-up visits. Decentration greater than 0.5 mm has also been reported in 43% of eyes implanted with the Iris Claw Lens.[1,12]

The greatest concern regarding modern anterior chamber phakic IOLs has been endothelial cell loss. Widely disparate results have been cited recently. Decreasing the haptic-optic angle and optic thickness in the ZBMF Baikoff lens has helped achieve better results, with average endothelial cell loss of approximately 4%.[12] In a detailed study comparing the Baikoff anterior chamber lens to the Worst Iris Claw Lens, Perez-Santoja et al. found similar average losses in mean endothelial cell density between the two groups. The Worst cohort had an average progressive endothelial cell loss of 13% at 12 months. A recent study of endothelial cell loss with this lens found endothelial cell reductions to slowly increase from 3.85% at 6 months to 13.4% at 4-year follow-up.[1]

POSTERIOR CHAMBER LENSES

Posterior Chamber Plate Haptic Lens

Posterior chamber plate haptic lenses (Chiron/Adatomed [Chiron Intraoptics, Boca Raton, FL], Staar Surgical [Staar, Monrovia, CA], International Vision [Cincinnati, OH]) are thin, one-piece, plate haptic structures designed to be placed in the posterior chamber between the iris and crystalline lens.[1] They are similar to posterior chamber plate lenses used for aphakia, but phakic plate lenses are thinner, longer, and more flexible.[1] The Staar lens is made of high refractive index collagen-hydrogel copolymer, whereas the Chiron lens is made of silicone. The haptics ride in the ciliary sulcus and resemble the Fyodorov model. The vault of the lens avoids contact with the zonular fibers and the crystalline lens capsule, leaving a space on ultrasonography of approximately 0.2 mm.[1]

Plate lenses are slightly easier to insert than Iris Claw Lenses, although great care is required not to touch the crystalline lens, because doing so could lead to anterior subcapsular lens opacity.[1]

The major unresolved issues with the posterior chamber plate lenses are potential for cataract formation, long-term stability of lens position, and the risk of chronic breakdown of the blood-aqueous barrier. The causes of the lens opacity are uncertain, but may include surgical trauma, metabolic disturbance, and intermittent contact between the IOL and crystalline lens.[1] The issue of late decentration requires further study of design features and necessitates innovative preoperative measurement techniques in sizing the lens. Long-term uveal contact is possible, increasing the risk of chronic inflammation because the lenses are not fixed firmly.[1]

Staar Implantable Contact Lens

The current Staar Surgical implantable contact lens (ICL) is made of porcine collagen/hydroxymethyl methacrylate (HEMA) copolymer with a refractive index of 1.45 at 35°C. The material is soft, elastic, and hydrophilic. The plate haptic design is a posterior chamber lens that is foldable and capable of being inserted through a 3-mm corneal incision under topical anesthesia (Figure 11.9). Available powers range from 3–20 D correction of myopia and 3–17 D correction of hyperopia. Currently, five lens lengths are manufactured ranging from 10.8–13.0 mm to accommodate different eye sizes. The optic portion measures 4.5–5.5 mm. The Staar Toric ICL is currently available in Europe.

Lens power determination is calculated using formulas developed by Feingold and Olsen. The independent variables include the following: pre-

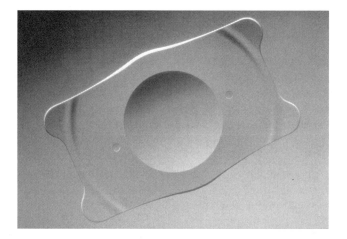

FIGURE 11.9. Staar Surgical Implantable Contact Lens (Staar Surgical, Monrovia, CA) is a plate lens inserted into the posterior chamber and is capable of being inserted through a 3-mm clear corneal incision. (Courtesy of Staar Surgical, Monrovia, CA.)

operative spheric equivalent, vertex distance, average keratometry, and actual anterior chamber depth. The final choice of lens power is determined by desired postoperative refraction, lens availability, and the surgeon's experience. The ICL length is based on the patient's corneal diameter. Generally, a lens that has a diameter of 0.5 mm more than the corneal diameter is implanted to promote proper ICL vaulting.[1,12] The lens rests on the anterior zonular fibers with the posterior surface being concave, vaulting over the anterior lens capsule of the crystalline lens to provide space for the aqueous.

Zaldivar found complications of implanting ICLs for myopia and hyperopia to include pupillary block, cataracts, and retinal detachment. Cataracts have been found to occur with an incidence rate between 1% and 10%, depending on surgical skill and experience, lens design, and lens sizing.[12] Lens sizing remains the crucial problem of phakic intraocular lens usage. Other complications include improper refractive result, decentration of the optic portion of the lens, and pigmentary glaucoma.

A lens that vaults with excessive apical clearance from being too large creates a spinnaker effect, resulting in significant undercorrection and a tendency to cause angle closure glaucoma. This type of glaucoma is a result of a lens that pushes the iris diaphragm forward. A lens that is too small may cause cataract formation. A white to white measurement + 0.5 mm has been advocated in determining proper lens size for implantation in phakic eyes. An incorrect sizing occurs in a high percentage of eyes (more than 50%). Apparently, there is so much variation in anatomic conformation of the eye that the correspondence to white to white and internal sulcus to sulcus measurements is often pure chance. The sulcus to sulcus distance can only be accurately measured with the aid of high frequency, high resolution ultrasound technology. To assure an adequate fit, other anatomic features must be taken into consideration. These features include anterior chamber depth and the radius of curvature of the surface of anterior crystalline lens. The anterior crystalline lens curvature is now being measured using the Scheimpflug camera. Generally, larger-size lenses (when compared to other one-piece IOL designs) are needed with a larger anterior chamber depth.

Adatomed (Chiron) Lens

The silicone material of the Adatomed lens (Chiron Intraoptics, Boca Raton, FL) is an elastomer with a refractive index of 1.41. The lens is large (6.5-mm width with a 5.5-mm optic zone) and long (11.0–13.5 mm) in 0.5-mm steps with a large optic zone. It is in contact with the anterior capsule of the crystalline lens. The lens is more difficult than most to insert and requires a 6-mm incision. This fixation may be the reason for reported cases of anterior capsular fibrosis. The edge of the optic zone is rather thin. Pigmentary dispersion has been reported by many investigators.[14] In 1996, Fechner et al. reported eight of 45 eyes implanted showed subcapsular opacity at 2 years postoperatively.[1] Marinho noted decentration in four of 40 eyes he implanted with the Adatomed lens.[1,9] The lens has been withdrawn from the market due to cataract formation, late decentration, and propensity for pigmentary glaucoma.

PC Posterior Refractive Lens

The PC posterior refractive lens is manufactured by International Vision (Cincinnati, OH) from silicone with a refractive index of 1.46. The diameter of the optic zone is 4.5–5.5 mm, depending on the optic power of the lens. The lens corrects for myopia and hyperopia and is soft, elastic, and hydrophilic. It is relatively easy to insert through a clear corneal incision of 3.0–3.5 mm. The lens appears to have no contact with the anterior lens capsule of the crystalline lens. No synechiae have been noted in follow-up. If necessary, it can be removed with little difficulty. The most common complication to date has been decentration, especially with earlier models that were smaller. Decentration appears to be directly related to the length of the optic. Power ranges include 6–22 D for the correction of myopia and 3–16 D for the correction of hyperopia. There must be adequate anterior chamber depth of approximately 2.75 mm or greater. Laser YAG iridectomies at 11 o'clock and 1 o'clock are recommended and are generally performed approximately 2 days or more before the intraocular surgery to eliminate the possibility of pupillary block.

A unilateral high myopic study in children is currently under way. The lens can be used instead of a contact lens or aniseikonic spectacle correction. The phakic intraocular lens can easily be removed or replaced. A scleral reinforcing surgery 1–2 months before implantation for the purpose of slowing growth of the eye can be performed.[14]

BIOPTIC CONCEPT

Zaldivar has introduced the concept termed *bioptic combination,* whereby any residual refractive error is corrected by LASIK at 1–3 months after posterior phakic lens implantation. Guell uses a similar procedure, except that the flap is created before insertion of an iris claw phakic lens to avoid endothelial-intraocular lens touch during the keratectomy. This adjustable refractive surgery technique is performed 1–3 months after the lens insertion into the anterior chamber.

FUTURE DIRECTIONS

Each of the anterior and posterior chamber phakic lenses has promise, but significant issues must be resolved before wide acceptance is gained. Problems with anterior chamber angle–supported phakic lenses are intermittent endothelial touch, rotation of the lens affecting the angle, ocular pain, ovalization of the pupil, and glare or halos.[1] Future lens designs will attempt to rectify these concerns. Iris-supported lenses are technically more difficult to implant and have long-term safety concerns relative to progressive endothelial loss, iris atrophy, and aqueous flare.

The major unresolved issues with posterior chamber phakic lenses are cataract formation, long-term stability of the lens position, and risk of chronic breakdown of the blood-aqueous barrier.[1] The causes of anterior subcapsular cataract formation are possibly due to surgical trauma, metabolic disturbances, or intermittent contact between the phakic lens and crystalline lens.[1,9,10] Accurate sizing of the lens remains an issue. Late decentration can be a result of inadequate sizing. Because the lenses are not fixed firmly, additional concerns are the chronic contact of the lens to uveal tissue and possible effects to the blood-aqueous barrier.

The preservation of visual axis, maintaining corneal asphericity, and accommodation achieved with the use of phakic intraocular lenses make this area of refractive surgery research quite attractive. These early lens designs appear to be relatively stable, somewhat predictable, and reversible, making them a viable option to patients with high ametropia. Although phakic intraocular lenses bring a new set of complications, many unresolved problems remain with corneal refractive procedures, especially in patients with high refractive errors.[1] With expected advances, phakic intraocular lenses are certain to gain additional attention of ophthalmic surgeons performing refractive surgery.

Clear Lens Extractions

In 1890, Fukala was the first to be given credit for advocating extraction of a clear lens to gain refractive correction.[1] Surgically induced retinal detachment was recognized as an early complication. Other complications of intraocular surgery include endophthalmitis, cystoid macular edema, glaucoma, and posterior capsular opacification. The key issue is the extent and risk of retinal detachment in axial myopes.[15-17] The incidence of retinal detachment in phakic patients appears to be 0.005–0.010%. An increase to 1.0–9.6% can be expected with the type of procedure expected in clear lens extraction.[1,14] Barraquer et al. found a twofold greater risk of retinal detachment in younger myopes who have clear lens extraction. The incidence is expected to increase over time. Lindstrom found a 5% incidence rate of retinal detachment at 5 years.[2] Retinal detachment surgery in axial myopes with thin sclera makes it more difficult to attach the retina in most cases. Critics point to articles that demonstrate an excessive risk of significant vision loss.[15] This is dramatically demonstrated in a report by Ripandelli et al. of 41 retinal detachments that occurred within 4 years of clear lens extraction.[17] Of operated eyes, 88% were successfully reattached, and only 22% of such eyes achieved a vision of 20/60 or better. In other studies on the repair of retinal detachment in axial myopes, up to 77% may be left with vision worse than 20/50. The incidence of posterior capsular opacification may be as high as 60%.[1]

With respect to hyperopia, more procedures are done worldwide for moderate to excessive hyperopia as accommodation wanes with age. An IOL is needed to correct for the aphakia rendered. The risk of postoperative retinal detachment is not increased as it is in myopia, but is similar to the rate found in emmetropia; however, it is important to identify nanophthalmic eyes because choroidal effusion and malignant glaucoma are significant operative risks.[1,15]

The technique is relatively straightforward. The preferred methods of extraction are small incision, extracapsular surgery, including phacoemulsification, and manual removal. Because the surgery is performed on a clear lens of a young patient with a bright reflex, wide pupillary dilatation, and soft nucleus, the surgery is simplified. The surgeon may choose to insert a foldable or two-piece polymethlymethacrylate IOL into the capsular bag. The possible loss of visibility that accompanies silicone lenses during vitrectomy with gas-fluid exchange or silicone oil may make it better to avoid silicone materials in this group.

Corneaplasty

Advanced Corneal Systems, along with Sandoz Pharmaceuticals, have conducted trials to reshape the cornea using hyaluronidase to alter the stroma by placing a contact lens on the front of the eye for a controlled contour effect. The enzyme temporarily breaks down proteoglycan bonds. The enzyme is injected by a needle patch that allows for a circular pattern to be applied to the cornea. This method uses the principles of orthokeratology.

Rigid lenses are worn initially for several hours a day. Stabilizing enzyme drops are administered while the lens is worn. The procedure can be repeated until the desired results are obtained. Studies evaluating safety and efficacy are currently being conducted and address such issues and concerns as predictability, stability, and reversibility.

Corneal Onlays

Synthetic keratophakia was first introduced by Barraquer to overcome the problems encountered with keratomileusis and keratophakia for the correction of aphakia.[1,18] Synthetic onlays were fraught with complications, including corneal acceptance (edema), vascularization, and necrosis. As with epikeratophakia, introduced by Kaufman, keratophakia is technically difficult to perform, unpredictable, and generally considered not to be entirely reversible. Keratophakia occurs when the onlay is sutured onto the corneal surface. One modification no longer used is epikeratophakia, in which a living tissue is reshaped and placed on the cornea. Although epikeratophakia may be generally considered to be a reversible procedure, it has virtually been abandoned because it is fraught with many similar complications. In addition, epikeratophakia requires lyophilized human donor tissue sutured to the donor cornea.[19]

Intracorneal Implants

The use of synthetic lenses for stromal implantation eliminates the problem of requiring donor tissue (availability, quality, damage during procedure with autografts).[20–22] Many materials have been used since Barraquer first used polymethylmethacrylate in 1949. Currently, two different synthetic materials for implantation exist: rigid polysulfone and soft hydrogel hydroxyethylmethacrylate.

Polysulfone Inlays

Polysulfone inlays have a high index of refraction (1.633) relative to the cornea, allowing a refractive effect to be produced when implanted into the cornea.[1] Polysulfone has several shortcomings, including its impermeable nature, but it does possess UV-absorbing qualities.[1,16,23] To achieve proper placement, a deep lamellar dissection must be performed to create a stromal pocket for lens placement.[1,23] Significant sight-threatening complications have been reported, including the following: stromal melt, visual axis opacity and scarring (Figure 11.10), Descemet's tears, incursion into the anterior chamber, wound dehiscence, neovascularization, and irregular astigmatism.[1,23] Fenestrations do not permit adequate permeability of nutrients to flow into or through the implant.[1] Concerns have been raised about obtaining accurate intraocular pressure readings and endothelial cell counts after corneal inlays.[20]

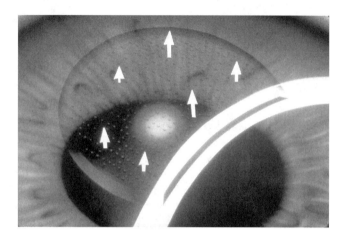

FIGURE 11.10. Schematic of a stromal lens showing the position of a synthetic inlay.

Hydrogel Lens Implants

Hydrogel material with a high water content is very permeable to nutrients. Because the material is of similar index of refraction compared to the cornea, it transmits its refractive effect through alteration of the anterior corneal surface by creating a bulge.[1,18] The refractive effect is in proportion to implant depth; therefore, if placed too deep into the cornea, little desired effect is accomplished.[1] A free cap is required, but Binder reported a reversible nature to this procedure.[20]

Larger-diameter lenses (6.75 mm versus 5.5 mm) produce less irregular astigmatism, and endothelial cell loss appears stable over time (7.5%). Lens manufacturing difficulties can cause lens impermeability, leading to corneal necrosis over the implant.[1,20]

Recently, a small diameter lens called the *SDICL* (Chiron Intraoptics, Boca Raton, FL) was investigated for the correction of myopia. Like polysulfone, the SDICL performs as a lens positioned as an intrastromal implant and provides adequate alterations of the anterior corneal surface.[1] Initial studies found the lens to be well tolerated and predictable; however, a number of concerns still exist. Complications occurred similar to other synthetic implants, including migration of the implant and corneal edema.[16–21]

Future Direction

The future of polysulfone and, to a lesser extent, hydrogel materials does not have a favorable outlook mainly due to the poor biocompatibility, stability, and predictability of implanting these materials into the stroma.[1,23] New synthetic materials may play a role in the future of refractive surgical techniques. A variety of lens designs have already been proposed for the correction of presbyopia and congenital and acquired disfigurements of the iris (aniridia, albinism, and other symptomatic iris anomalies).[18]

INTRACORNEAL RING SEGMENTS

Intracorneal ring segments (ICRS), or *Intacs* (KeraVision, Fremont, CA), are made of polymethylmethacrylate and two segments are inserted into the peripheral stroma of the cornea for myopia at two-thirds of depth. The effect is achieved based on increased device thickness. There is a limited reshaping effect to maintain a similar asphericity of the cornea (prolate versus oblate) with this procedure; therefore, the limited range of correction is possible with ICRS. Currently, three segment thicknesses are approved: 0.25, 0.3, and 0.35 that correct 1.3 D, 2 D, and 2.7 D of myopia, respectively. Clinical trials have begun on 0.21-, 0.4-, and 0.45-thickness segments with hope of correcting up to 4 D of myopia (Figure 11.11).[24]

This procedure offers three major advantages: It is removable or exchangeable, it does not involve the visual axis, and it maintains corneal asphericity. If the patient has an adverse effect, such as an increase in astigmatism, the segments simply can be removed. Clinical studies to date have shown that 82% of patients with removed Intacs return to within 0.5 D of their original refractive error. If the patient is over- or undercorrected, an exchange to a thicker or thinner segment may be performed. By only involving the peripheral cornea in the surgical procedure, there is less risk of a loss of best corrected visual acuity. By viewing a topographic or Orbscan image, it is evident that the same prolate pattern is present in eyes

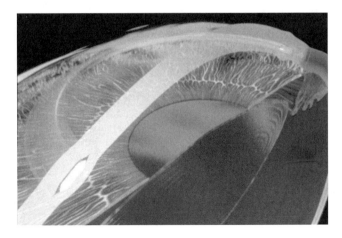

FIGURE 11.11. Schematic showing the position of ring segments from KeraVision used for the correction of myopia. (Courtesy of KeraVision, Fremont, CA.)

after Intacs (Figure 11.12). But we may also be able to see the effect of a positive asphericity when we compare the ICRS in Phase III to LASIK. Two groups of patients 4 D and under with less than 1 D of astigmatism were studied (Table 11.1). The same surgeon, Daniel S. Durrie, performed both types of procedures, and no enhancements were allowed in either procedure. Looking at predictability (Figure 11.13) in the ± 1-D range, the two are fairly comparable, with 92% of the LASIK patients and 90% of ICRS patients refracting to ± 1 D of intended. With 79% of LASIK patients and 76% of the ICRS patients refracting to ± 0.5 D, this shows no statistically significant difference.[25]

When examining visual acuity of 20/20 or better, we see a significant difference. The number of patients uncorrected at 20/20 or better after

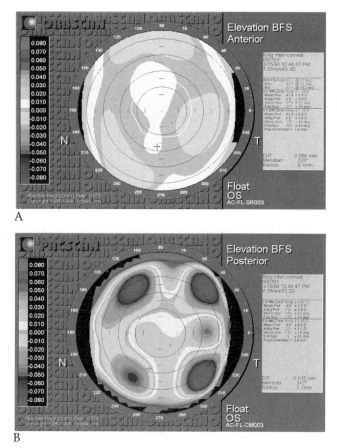

A

B

FIGURE 11.12. Postoperative anterior (**A**) and posterior (**B**) elevation after the placement of Intacs (ring segments) for myopia.

TABLE 11.1
ICRS Phase III vs. LASIK

---

50 eyes ICRS Phase III
    Myopia: –4.00 to –1.00 D
    No enhancements
    Single surgeon
46 eyes CRS LASIK Study
    Myopia: –4.00 to –1.00 D
    Summit Apex Plus laser
    No enhancements
    Single surgeon

CRS = Casebeer Reynolds Study; ICRS = intracorneal ring segments.

LASIK was 68% compared to 82% for the ICRS. Twenty-seven percent were 20/16 or better with LASIK, and 63% were 20/16 or better with ICRS. This substantial difference is likely due to maintaining the corneal asphericity and central vision.

    Overall, the Intacs procedures show potential but, as with all refractive surgery procedures, patient selection is a critical part of whether it will be successful.

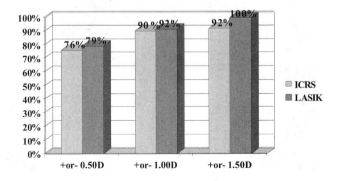

FIGURE 11.13. Comparable predictability is shown with Intacs versus LASIK correction. (ICRS = intracorneal ring segments.)

INTACS FOR HYPEROPIA

The latest development for Intacs is a procedure for hyperopia. The peripheral cornea is again involved, but unlike the segments for myopia, there are six smaller segments rather than two. They are inserted in a radial fashion as shown at two-thirds the depth of the cornea. They work by shortening the arc length in the region they are placed. Because the angle is toward the limbus, these smaller segments shorten the peripheral arc length, causing the central cornea to steepen, the corneal radius to shorten, and subsequent elimination of hyperopia (Figure 11.14).

A study was performed by Dr. Arturo S. Chayet in Tijuana, Mexico, using six segments of 1.5–2.0 mm in length on 17 patients with a mean age of 47.6 years. The preoperative refractive errors ranged from +1 to +4 D, with a mean refractive error of +2.47. The 1-month postoperative results showed 81% of patients at 20/40 or better, 50% at 20/25 or better, and 31% at 20/20 or better. By 6 months, the visual acuity had improved to 100% at 20/40 or better, 93% at 20/25 or better, and 71% at 20/20 or better. No patients had a loss of best corrected visual acuity, and three patients actually gained a line in best corrected visual acuity.[25]

Another study, involving 1.8-mm segments on 14 patients, showed even more impressive results at 1 month postoperatively. Using these six 1.8-mm segments, 100% of patients were 20/40 or better, 92% were 20/25 or better, and 85% were 20/20 or better. Of the 14 eyes treated, nine gained

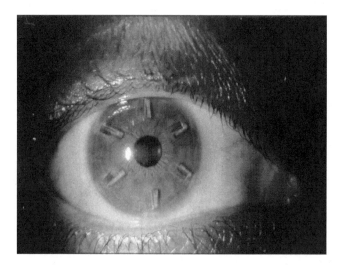

FIGURE 11.14. Hyperopic Intacs are small segments implanted in a radial fashion to steepen the central cornea. (Courtesy of KeraVision, Fremont, CA.)

a line in best corrected visual acuity, and there was no reported loss in best corrected visual acuity. Although clinical trials are just preparing to begin in the United States, the international data suggest another potential procedure to improve the lives of hyperopic patients.

As these new procedures develop and discussion of a prototype for astigmatism correction using Intacs proceeds, the addition of implants and inlays may gain patient acceptance. Its peripheral surgical location, as well as its ability to be removed, make acceptance inevitable.

Presbyopia

Surgical correction of presbyopia has been under investigation for a number of years and has received special attention recently as the generation of baby boomers enter their early to mid-40s. By changing our thinking regarding why presbyopia occurs, we have opened the doors for two surgical techniques that propose to restore accommodation: anterior ciliary sclerotomy and scleral expansion. Laser modification of the crystalline lens for presbyopia is also under investigation. The surgical approaches currently performed worldwide are considered compensatory approaches and fall under the category of either monovision or multifocal correction.[1] Techniques used for monovision correction include LTK, PRK, and LASIK. Multifocal approaches have been achieved through both corneal procedures and the use of specialized IOLs in both phakic eyes and after lens extraction.

SCLERAL EXPANSION AND ANTERIOR CILIARY SCLEROTOMY

Schachar developed a theory of accommodation that focuses on the diameter of the crystalline lens changing during accommodation.[26] This was demonstrated in vitro and in vivo, as well as with the theoretic lens model. Schachar et al. state that as the lens is comprised of ectodermal tissue and continues to grow through the course of life, the working distance between the ciliary body and the crystalline lens must decrease as a person ages.[1,26] This shortened distance decreases the effectiveness of the ciliary body on the equator of the lens as it attempts to increase lens diameter, resulting in presbyopia. Anterior ciliary sclerotomy is one of the surgical techniques based on Schachar's premise. In this surgery, radial incisions in the anterior sclera are made to assist the ciliary body increase lens diameter. Scleral expansion is a surgical technique in which the ciliary body is expanded through the insertion of a synthetic band posterior to the limbus that stretches the sclera (Figure 11.15). These two surgical techniques are currently under clinical investigation.

Contradicting Schachar's theory and procedural success, Mathews conducted a study on presbyopes after scleral expansion surgery using a dynamic infrared optometer to record accommodation levels. He concluded

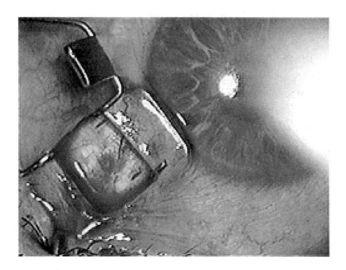

FIGURE 11.15. Scleral expansion through the insertion of a synthetic band anterior to the limbus has been used to improve accommodation in presbyopes. (Courtesy of Richard W. Yee, http://eye.med.uth.tmc.edu/RWYee/presby.htm)

that because there was no true restoration of accommodation after the surgery, another reason—possibly memorization, better blur interpretation, or simply encouragement—must explain why the subjects read smaller near letters postoperatively.[26]

PHOTOPHAKO REDUCTION AND PHOTOPHAKO MODULATION

Treatment of the clear crystalline lens with a laser to correct presbyopia has been proposed by Myers and Krueger.[27] This technique is based on the hypothesis that presbyopia is caused by lens growth–induced volume changes, lens mass distribution changes, and reduction in lens flexure. The first proposed method is called *photophako reduction* and entails reducing lens volume. The second modifies such lens properties as flexure and nutrient transport and is called *photophako modulation* (PPM). Photoablation or photodisruption of the crystalline lens would be achieved through a low-powered, focused, and scanning laser that restores accommodation by either selective reduction of lens volume (cavitation) or by softening the nucleus (microperforation). Photophako reduction would involve an annular treatment pattern about the visual axis to change the angle of zonular insertion with volume reduction and geometric lens changes.[27] Microperforations in photophako modulation in the peripheral lens nucleus could modify flexure without causing light scatter and cataractogenesis.[27]

The Nd:YLF picosecond laser has been shown to successfully photo-disrupt the lens in rabbit studies without causing cataract formation. The goal would be to treat people 35–45 years of age with the Nd:YLF laser and restore from 5 to 8 D of accommodation, postponing presbyopia for 8–10 years. Other factors that must be considered involve the beam's traversing the cornea and aqueous without being absorbed. Laser modification of the crystalline lens to correct presbyopia has become a hot topic in the refractive surgery industry and will be under investigation in the years to come.[27]

Monovision Techniques

Monovision techniques to treat hyperopia, or even emmetropia, and to induce myopia in a presbyopic eye have been used with mild to moderate success over the past few years. LASIK, PRK, and LTK are the procedures of choice for compensatory presbyopic surgery. These procedures offer the preservation of best spectacle-corrected visual acuity and contrast sensitivity while reducing stereopsis and uncorrected distance acuity in the surgical eye (see Chapter 3, Monovision and LASIK). Jain et al. performed a systematic review of published literature regarding monovision success and visual outcomes.[28] Some pertinent findings included a mean success rate of 73%, less than 50 seconds of arc stereoacuity reduction, as well as a minimal reduction of binocular visual acuity and depth of focus. At spatial frequencies higher than four cycles per degree, binocular contrast sensitivity function was significantly reduced.[28]

Multifocal Correction

In multifocal correction, PRK, LASIK, radial keratotomy, and intracorneal lenses have been used to treat presbyopic myopes with preservation of binocularity. Bauerberg proposes performing inferior off-center ablation with LASIK for the correction of both hyperopia and presbyopia. Early results have shown this procedure to offer better distance and near acuity than centered ablation.[29] Zonal PRK with a specially designed mask treating approximately 15% of a 3-mm pupil may be another procedure with a promising future for surgical presbyopic correction.[30] Implanting a multifocal IOL theoretically offers an excellent balance of distance and near vision, but its drawbacks include increased risk of retinal problems, infection, necessity for precision placement, and loss of approximately one line of best spectacle-corrected visual acuity with decreased contrast sensitivity.

Conclusions

A shift in correcting high refractive errors from extraocular corneal reshaping to extraocular phakic and stromal implant investigational procedures has occurred. This shift is due mainly to the functional and anatomic limitations of corneal flattening techniques. Some of the very same concepts performed years ago by pioneers including Baraquer, Kaufman, and Kelman are being revisited as potentially viable options in correcting refractive errors today. Many of these procedures are already familiar to most ophthalmic surgeons.

Careful scrutiny of current technology and creative innovations will undoubtedly allow for the possibility of someday correcting all forms of refractive error, especially those that are most disabling. Extensive research in the areas of enhanced vision correction beyond 20/20 and the successful management of presbyopia will continue to attract much interest in the specialty of refractive surgery.

References

1. Friedman NJ, Husain SE, Kohnen T, Koch DD. Investigational Refractive Procedures. In M Yanoff (ed), Ophthalmology. Philadelphia: Mosby, 1999;7.1–7.16.
2. Karpecki PM. Beyond topography guided ablation. Rev Optom 1999;136:115–116.
3. Koch DD, Kohnen T, McDonnell PJ, Menefee RF, Berry MJ. Hyperopia correction by non-contact holmium:YAG laser thermal keratoplasty, United States phase IIA clinical study with a 1-year follow-up. Ophthalmology 1996;103:1532–1535.
4. Singer H. Studies show Ho:YAG LTK for hyperopia, presbyopia effective and safe. Ocular Surg News 1999;17(14):10–2.
5. Brown D. Laser thermokeratoplasty: A new tool for refractive surgeons and comprehensive ophthalmologists. J Cataract Refract Surg 1999;3:1,33–34.
6. Kohl M. Eyes remain stable after RFK, studies show. Ocular Surg News 1999;18:49–53.
7. Femto Group, Institute of Applied Physics, University of Heidelberg, www.aphys.uni-heidelberg.de/AG_Bille/Projekt/femto.html. Accessed October 16, 1999.
8. Krueger R. The picosecond laser for non-mechanical laser in situ keratomileusis. J Refract Surg 1998;14:467–469.
9. Praeger DL. Innovations and creativity in contemporary ophthalmology: preliminary experience with the phakic myopic intraocular lens. Ann Ophthalmol 1988;20:456–462.
10. Waring GO, Alleman N, Baikoff G, et al. Refractive Symposium: Phakic IOLs—setting the standard. Presented at the Society of Cataract and Refractive Surgery, Seattle, 1996.
11. Koch DD. Enter with caution (editorial). J Cataract Refractive Surg 1996;22:153–154.
12. Baikoff G. The place of refractive IOLs in the treatment of high myopia. ISRS Conference, Atlanta, 1995.
13. Probst L. Phakic intraocular lenses. NECO Conference. Boston, 1999.

14. Rozakis, G. History of PRLs. Second International Course On Phakic Refractive Lenses For the Posterior Chamber. Milano, Italy, 1999.
15. Buratto L. Considerations on clear lens extraction in high myopia. Eur J Implant Ref Surg 1991;3:221–226.
16. Goldberg MF. Clear lens extraction for axial myopia: an appraisal. Ophthalmol 1987;94:571–582.
17. Ripandelli G, Billi B, Fedelli R, Stripe IV. Retinal detachment after clear lens extraction in patients with high myopia. Retina 1996;16:3–6.
18. Aquavella JA, Shovlin JP, DePaolis MD. Contact Lenses and Refractive Surgery. In M Harris (ed), Problems In Optometry. Philadelphia: JB Lippincott, 1990.
19. Werblin TP, Peiffer RI, Patel AS. Synthetic keratophakia for the correction of aphakia. Ophthalmol 1987;94:926–934.
20. Binder PS, Zavalla EY, Deg JK, Baumgartner SD. Alloplastic implants for the correction of refractive errors. Ophthalmol 1984;91:806–814.
21. Parks RA, McCarey BE. Hydrogel keratophakia: long term morphology in the monkey model. CLAO J 1991;17:216–222.
22. Weberlin TP, Patel AS. Myopic hydrogel keratophakia: Improvements in lens design. Cornea 1987;6:197–201.
23. Lane SL, Lindstrom RI, Williams PA, Lindstrom CW. Polysulfone intracorneal lenses. J Refract Corneal Surg 1985;1:207–216.
24. Burris TE, Baker PC, Ayer CT, et al. Flattening of the central corneal curvature with intrastromal rings of increasing thickness: an eye-bank eye study. J Cataract Refract Surg 1993;19:182–187.
25. Durrie DS, Asbell PA, Burris TE. Reversible refractive effect: data from phase II study of the 360 degree ICR in myopic eyes. Presented at the American Society of Cataract and Refractive Surgery, Seattle, 1996.
26. Mathews S. Scleral expansion surgery does not restore accommodation in human presbyopia. Ophthalmology 1999;106:873–877.
27. Myers R, Krueger R. Novel approaches to correction of presbyopia with laser modification of the crystalline lens. J Refractive Surg 1998;14:136–139.
28. Jain S, Arora I, Azar DT. Success of monovision in presbyopes: review of the literature and potential applications to refractive surgery. Surv Ophthalmol 1996;40:491–499.
29. Bauerberg JM. Centered vs. inferior off-center ablation to correct hyperopia and presbyopia. J Refractive Surg 1999;15:66–69.
30. Vinciguerra P, Nizzola GM, Bailo G, et al. Excimer laser PRK for presbyopia: 24-month follow-up in three eyes. J Refractive Surg 1998;14:31–37.

Index

Note: Entries followed by *t* indicate tables; entries followed by *f* indicate figures.